Health and Well-Being across the Life Course

15 MAR 2024

SAGE has been part of the global academic community since 1965, supporting high quality research and learning that transforms society and our understanding of individuals, groups and cultures. SAGE is the independent, innovative, natural home for authors, editors and societies who share our commitment and passion for the social sciences.

Find out more at: **www.sagepublications.com**

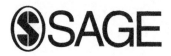

Health and Well-Being across the Life Course

Mary Larkin

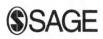

Los Angeles | London | New Delhi
Singapore | Washington DC

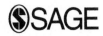

Los Angeles | London | New Delhi
Singapore | Washington DC

SAGE Publications Ltd
1 Oliver's Yard
55 City Road
London EC1Y 1SP

SAGE Publications Inc.
2455 Teller Road
Thousand Oaks, California 91320

SAGE Publications India Pvt Ltd
B 1/I 1 Mohan Cooperative Industrial Area
Mathura Road
New Delhi 110 044

SAGE Publications Asia-Pacific Pte Ltd
3 Church Street
#10-04 Samsung Hub
Singapore 049483

Editor: Sarah Gibson
Assistant editor: Emma Milman
Production editor: Katie Forsythe
Marketing manager: Tamara Navaratnam
Typeset by: C&M Digitals (P) Ltd, Chennai, India
Printed by MPG Books Group, Bodmin, Cornwall

First published 2013

Library of Congress Control Number: 2012941837

British Library Cataloguing in Publication data

A catalogue record for this book is available from
the British Library

MIX
Paper from
responsible sources
FSC® C018575

ISBN 978-0-85702-881-5
ISBN 978-0-85702-882-2 (pbk)

This book is dedicated to a true life course friend, Molly Brewer Hoeg

Contents

About the Author

Dr Mary Larkin is a Principal Lecturer in the Faculty of Health and Life Sciences at De Montfort University, Leicester. She is also Programme Leader for the BA Health Studies and BSc Public and Community Health. She has published widely in her main research areas of health and well-being and health and social care.

Introduction

Overview

- Aims and rationale of the book
- Chapter outlines
- Chapter features

Aims and Rationale of the Book

The terms 'health and well-being' and 'the life course' have featured more and more frequently in research and literature about age and ageing in recent years. Indeed, there is now an established body of knowledge on health and well-being at particular stages in our lives. The 'life course approach' has been used to supplement biological- and epidemiological-based explanations of health and well-being and has gained in credibility over the past decade. As a result, it has been increasingly adopted within a variety of disciplines and is now widely accepted as a contemporary theoretical framework. The growth in the acknowledgement that adverse health effects are cumulative from conception, through to infancy, childhood, adolescence, adulthood and old age is one of the main drivers behind these developments. The political commitment to preventing ill health by promoting healthy living at all ages to lay the foundations for better health throughout the life course also reflects the extent to which the life course perspective has been applied to policy and practice.

The main aim of this book is to synthesise the existing body of national and international literature on health and well-being across all of the life stages and the life course approach into one text and to provide the reader with a comprehensive and contemporary account of health and well-being across the whole lifespan from a life course perspective. It will do this by addressing key issues associated with health and well-being during each stage of the life course and will cover prenatal influences on health, and the health and well-being of children, adolescents, young adults, those who are middle-aged and older people. The material presented will be interpreted from a life course perspective in order to illustrate the extent to which health effects can accumulate across the various stages of the life course. Relevant policy initiatives will also be evaluated and any implications for future policy and practice highlighted. An eclectic approach will be adopted with regards to the disciplines that will be drawn on and these will include epidemiology, public health, health policy, medical sociology, the sociology of health and illness, social policy, social work, youth work, community studies and nursing.

Consequently, the book will meet the need for knowledge on an extensive range of courses about health and well-being at different life stages from the most recent perspective to achieve academic, political and practice-based currency – namely, the life course perspective. It is intended to be a core and/or supplementary text for first, second and third year students on undergraduate courses related to health, health and social care, working with children and young people, and childhood and adolescent studies as well as community work. Students taking pre- and post-registration courses in nursing and post-qualifying courses in social work will also find it useful. Furthermore, this book is ideal for students when they need to revisit their understanding of particular aspects of the subject areas that it addresses at different stages of, and on different modules on, their undergraduate studies. It has ongoing practical relevance and, as the reference list testifies, it contains a wealth of information about research and policy development from many sources that to date have not been drawn together in one volume. Therefore practitioners will also find the book invaluable for reference purposes. In addition, its content and pedagogical features will enable lecturers to use relevant chapters as a teaching resource to support and reinforce student learning.

As mentioned above, the body of literature on health and well-being in each of the main life stages is now more extensive and its growth looks set to continue. However, information and material is time-consuming to research because it is currently only available from numerous disparate sources and organisations. Therefore, the chapters in this book will draw on the wide range of contemporary literature about each of the stages and the reference list should be a resource in itself. Much relevant research is also being carried out in other Western countries, such as Australia, America and within member states of the European Union. Hence, whilst the emphasis will be on the United Kingdom, as the research emerging from these countries is highly applicable within the context of the United Kingdom both national and international literature will be used. Furthermore, the material presented and discussed will be located in its historical, European and wider international context as and when appropriate. Therefore, in addition to being suitable for its audience in the United Kingdom, the book also has relevance to Westernised Euro-American and Australasian audiences.

Chapter Outlines

Each of the main chapters will focus on health and well-being during one stage of the life course. These life stages will be loosely defined to acknowledge the fluid approach within the life course approach to categorisation by age. The chapters can be read independently or sequentially. Whatever their chosen usage of the book, readers are strongly advised to familiarise themselves with the key concepts and theories integral to the exploration of health and well-being across the life course discussed in Chapter 1 before starting any of the other chapters. All of the chapter headings, together with a brief outline of the content of each chapter, are set out below.

Chapter 1 Studying Health and Well-Being across the Life Course

This first chapter will provide readers with the relevant understandings that they require before engaging with other chapters in the book. It introduces several key concepts and theories and clarifies issues integral to any exploration of health and well-being in relation to the life course. These are: 'health and well-being', the 'life course', the life course perspective in general and more specifically, and the life course perspective on health and well-being. The varying patterns of mental and physical well-being over the life course will also be explored.

Chapter 2 Beginnings: Prenatal Health

The main focus of this chapter will be on the risks to an individual's health and well-being before birth. It will address the findings to date about pre-pregnancy and prenatal risks, together with the implications of these risks to the fetus and health and well-being across the life course. The debates and evidence about the extent to which these risks do compromise health and well-being in the longer term will also be considered. These discussions will include other factors that can be influential in modifying their effects.

Chapter 3 Health and Well-Being in Childhood

This chapter focuses on children from birth up to the beginning of their second decade. It starts by analysing data about the health and well-being of children in general in the United Kingdom, highlighting improvements and new health problems that have been identified. Health and well-being and childhood is then examined from a life course perspective. This involves an analysis of the ways in which it is shaped by prenatal influences, risks in childhood itself as well as the risks to future health that can occur during childhood. Other factors that are influential on children's health and well-being are also explored, as is the growth in the recognition of the effectiveness of a life course approach to health and well-being at policy level at this life stage.

Chapter 4 Health and Well-Being in Adolescence

The main adolescent health and well-being issues that are currently of particular concern is the first topic to be addressed in this chapter. It then explores the known factors that are likely to compromise health and well-being in adolescence from a life course perspective. This exploration includes a discussion of variables that modify the effects of these factors in different contexts. The chapter ends with a brief overview of the policies that have been developed to address issues around adolescent health and well-being in order to optimise health and well-being over a lifetime.

Chapter 5 Health and Well-Being in Young Adulthood

After defining young adulthood as the third and fourth decades of our lives, we will consider the arguments that this is one of the healthiest times of life and, overall, the healthiest stage of adulthood. The first part of the chapter looks at the effects of pregnancy, prenatal, childhood and adolescent influences on health and well-being in young adulthood. It then discusses the possible risks to health and well-being during young adulthood, and the extent to which these, alone and in combination with risk factors in preceding life stages, impact on health and well-being in middle and old age. The influences on the factors that can compromise health and well-being in young adulthood are addressed in the penultimate section. An overview of the policies that have been aimed at improving health and well-being in young adulthood is presented in the final section of the chapter.

Chapter 6 Health and Well-Being in Midlife

The term 'midlife' is currently used in relation to the period between the ages of 40 and 65. Although it is one of the least researched life stages, the literature available allows a comprehensive examination of health and well-being in middle adulthood from a life course perspective. After an overview of health and well-being during midlife, the chapter presents the findings from the discussions in the previous chapters about the effects of prenatal influences and exposure to risks during pregnancy, childhood, adolescence and young adulthood on health and well-being in midlife. This is followed by an exploration of possible risks to health and well-being during midlife and how these can also have implications for old age. A life course approach to health and well-being also requires an analysis of how these combine with other variables, such as risk factors from the preceding life stages and both negative *and* positive influences on the risks to health and well-being in midlife. Therefore, the next section presents such an analysis, together with any outcomes for health and well-being in midlife that have been identified. The chapter ends with a reflection on themes in recent policy initiatives aimed at improving health and well-being in midlife.

Chapter 7 Health and Well-Being in Old Age

This chapter provides a life course analysis of the complexity of the health and well-being of those over the age of 65. It starts with the main changes in health and well-being that occur during old age and the way that these are often accompanied by poor health and well-being. This is followed by an exploration of the cumulative risks and experiences from all of the preceding life stages. The risks to the health and well-being of older people and the way in which they increase and accumulate throughout old age are then discussed. The last two sections of the chapter address factors that can influence the outcomes of these risks, and policy initiatives that have attempted to make old age 'successful' and 'active'.

Chapter Features

The emphasis will be on explaining rather than assuming knowledge, and on making the text as accessible and interactive as possible. Features will include:

- an overview of each chapter
- an outline of the content and structure of each chapter
- key concepts will be highlighted in the text the first time that they are used and they are clearly outlined in the Glossary at the end of the book. The Glossary will provide relevant understandings for those with differing levels of knowledge. Its comprehensive nature means that it can also be used independently for reference purposes across a range of other modules and courses
- activities based on the text and on extracts from primary sources (for example, case studies, historical documents, newspaper articles, policy documents and statistical data). Where appropriate, post-activity comments to help the reader reflect on his/her work on the activities will be set out at the end of the chapters. Some of the activities can also be used and adopted by lecturers and tutors for workshops and classroom discussions. The presentation of these activities will be designed to reinforce and support students' learning as opposed to being essential to the main text in each chapter. They will be easily identified as they are presented in boxes and can be omitted by those students who do not require them
- links with other chapters will be highlighted
- tables, diagrams and graphs
- discussion points for either individual study or teaching purposes
- suggestions for further study and reading, plus Web resources

1

Studying Health and Well-Being across the Life Course

Overview

- Introduction
- 'Health and well-being'
- 'Life course'
- The life course perspective
- The life course and health and well-being
- The life course perspective on health and well-being
- Conclusions
- Summary
- Further study
- Activity comments

Introduction

As explained in the Introduction, there are certain concepts and theories that are central to an exploration of health and well-being across the life course. The two main concepts are 'health and well-being' and the 'life course'. Although other theories will be drawn on in different chapters in the book, the life course perspective on health and well-being is the theoretical approach that has the most relevance. Therefore the first part of this chapter will address 'health and well-being' and the 'life course'. In order to help you gain a full understanding about the life course approach to health and well-being, it will then introduce you to the life course perspective in general and the nature of the relationship between our life course and health and well-being. The last section of the chapter discusses the life course perspective on health and well-being itself, together with its various applications.

'Health and Well-Being'

Since the 1970s, there has been a move away from what is referred to as the **biomedical approach to health**. This approach draws heavily on scientific knowledge in general, and rests on the assumption that all causes of disease – mental disorders as well as physical conditions – can be understood in biological terms. Disease and sickness are therefore explained in terms of their specific or multiple causes, tracking the cause and the course of disease as it affects particular parts of the human body. In addition, disease and sickness are viewed as deviations from normal functioning. Hence, the biomedical approach sees health largely in mechanical terms, as a state where all parts of the body function 'normally' and there is an 'absence of disease'.

One of the outcomes of the decline of biomedicine within health **discourses** is that there has been a growing recognition that health is not solely determined by biological factors and that there are a multitude of influences that need to be taken into consideration when talking about health. Examples of these influences are psychological, environmental, social, economic and global factors. Consequently, during the last 50 years, broader approaches to health have been adopted. This was first encapsulated in the World Health Organization's (WHO) definition of health in 1946:

> Health is a state of complete physical, mental and social well-being, not merely the absence of disease or infirmity. (WHO, 1946: 100)

Subsequent definitions have continued to progress the move away from the narrow focus on 'scientific' biological conceptions of health in the biomedical discourse. For example:

> to reach a state of complete physical, mental and social well-being, an individual or group must be able to identify and realise aspirations, to satisfy needs, and to change or cope with the environment. Health is therefore seen as a resource for everyday life, not the objective of living. Health is a positive concept, emphasising social and personal resources, as well as physical capacities. (WHO, 1986: 1)

As the references to 'well-being', health as a 'resource for everyday life' and 'a positive concept' in these definitions indicate, not only is there now a more holistic approach to health but there is also a recognition that it is multidimensional

(Larkin, 2011a). Over the past decade, there has been a growing emphasis both nationally and internationally on one of these dimensions of health in particular – namely, 'well-being'. Indeed, the term 'health and well-being' as opposed to 'health' now features in the literature on health and illness across several disciplines (for example, psychology and economics) and is also used at a political level (Eckersley, 2009; Department of Health, 2010b). The introduction of 'Health and Wellbeing Boards' as part of the drive to improve health and care services and the health and well-being of local people from 2013 is further evidence of the extent of the adoption of this term (Department of Health, 2011b). However, there is a lack of consensus about the meaning of 'health and well-being'. This can be attributed to the fact that in addition to the multifaceted nature of 'health', 'well-being' is a complex and subjective concept that defies precise definition. This is evidenced by the way in which it varies between cultures and the fact that studies use different indicators in their attempts to measure it accurately. Moreover, there are different types of 'well-being', such as social, emotional and psychological well-being. As contrasting pictures of 'well-being' have emerged from the different measures used and from studies in different countries, the validity of the operationalisation of the concept of 'well-being' has been also criticised (Diener et al., 2003; Bradshaw and Mayhew, 2005; Blanchflower and Oswald, 2008; Eckersley, 2009).

Despite the absence of a definitive understanding of 'health and well-being', it is most commonly used to convey the idea that an important component of our general 'health' is our feelings about ourselves as human beings, our lives and our relationships. These feelings include our levels of happiness, the extent to which we feel a sense of fulfilment, and how satisfied we are with our lives. Although this book will be drawing on a wide range of literature that reflects the varying interpretations of 'health and well-being', as there is not a more sustainable definition the emphasis throughout the chapters will be on this more general usage.

'Life Course'

Since the 1980s, the concept of the 'life course' has gradually replaced that of the 'life cycle' within academic disciplines such as sociology, psychology and anthropology. This reflects the growing recognition that our lives are not divided into well-defined stages such as 'childhood', 'adulthood' and 'old age'. Moreover, the concept of the 'life cycle' itself has been criticised for being too deterministic because it does not acknowledge historical changes, cultural diversity and individual agency. Such criticisms have in part been fuelled by the evidence that 'age' has different meanings between cultures and across time; for example studies have shown that in foraging societies there is minimal social differentiation in terms of age (Vincent, 2003; Hunt, 2005). The literature on 'age' has also shown how age categories have varied historically. For instance, childhood in medieval Europe was not a distinct stage of life in that children were not regarded as significantly different from adults. They were integrated into adult working and social life, treated and dressed as miniature adults who gradually assumed adult roles as they matured into adulthood. Children in the lower classes worked at a very early age and for the same long hours as adults (Aries, 1965).

Some of these criticisms have been challenged. With reference to Aries's work on childhood, there are debates about the extent to which children were really integrated into the adult world. These debates focus on the way in which children were still viewed as being subordinate within the patriarchal and feudal social order of preindustrial societies. Furthermore, Aries's construction of childhood is not universal as in many Third World countries young children still work, often in very demanding circumstances. In addition, the fact that children are not passive actors and construct their own everyday reality should not be ignored (Jackson and Scott, 2006). Nonetheless, there has been a growing emphasis on cultural and historical variations in experiences of the different stages over the past two decades. Consequently, the view that stages in life are prescribed and predictable has been discredited and the validity of the arguments that these stages are **socially constructed** through a range of social, cultural, political and economic processes has been increasingly accepted (Hareven, 1995; Hunt, 2005; Vera-Sanso, 2006). Hence, the concept of an age-determined 'life cycle' has been eclipsed by the concept of 'life course' in which 'age' is essentially socially constructed.

Rapid sociocultural transformation is now a hallmark of contemporary societies. Examples of factors identified as being highly influential are globalisation, ever advancing technology, consumerism and demographic changes (Hunt, 2005; Green, 2010). The adoption of the broader concept of the 'life course' means that the impact of such important factors can be appropriately acknowledged in the interpretation of our life stages. For instance, there are concerns in the West that childhood is being eroded and that the boundaries between adulthood and childhood are becoming blurred. The move to the concept of the 'life course' has meant that explanations of this phenomenon now have increased their credibility. This is because, when identifying its underlying causes (such as precocious sexuality), they now consider key technological and social developments (such as the ease with which children now have access to adult information and adult lives) and mass conspicuous consumption.

Discussion Point

What are the arguments for and against the use of the concept of the 'life course' instead of the 'life cycle'?

The Life Course Perspective

This interest in the 'life course' spurred on the development of new theoretical perspectives. The life course perspective arose out of the confluence of several theoretical approaches and is the one that has achieved the most recognition during the past two decades (Hunt, 2005). Although there are different approaches within the life course perspective, a predominant theme is that stages in life are not necessarily standardised, chronologically or biologically fixed, sequential or gendered but are subject to a variety of social, historical and cultural influences. As a result, there is a 'ragged relationship between chronological age and life course categories' (Hockey and James, 2003: 63) without clear-cut and compulsory transitions between ages and life stages. Therefore, this perspective refutes temporal irreversibility and linearity in the life course. A range of evidence is cited in support of this refutation. Much of this evidence centres around the fluidity of the life course as demonstrated by the changing relationship between age and marriage in Western societies since the 1970s. This means that the average age of marriage is now later and childbearing is delayed. The persistence of youthful identities across several phases of the life course in contemporary society is another example of fluidity in the life course. Other evidence includes the way in which some life stages can recur, for instance through remarriage. The reconstruction of the life course over time as a result of the emergence of new life stages that are not just based on biological differentiation but are socially constructed through the cumulative effects of 'socio-economic and cultural changes' (Hareven, 1995: 132) is also used to argue that the life course is fluid. These new stages are childhood (as discussed above), adolescence, adulthood, engagement, homeownership, parenthood, grandparenthood and old age. In addition, evidence about the role of choice and agency and the extent to which individuals both negotiate their own life courses and shape their life trajectories is integral to theorising about the fluidity of the life course within this perspective (Cohen, 1987; Hareven, 1995; Hockey and James, 2003; Platt, 2011).

The argument within the life course perspective that the blurring of the relationship between age and identifiable life stages is in part due to the emergence of new life stages is nowhere more clearly illustrated than in its account of old age. In this account, the life course perspective identifies the sources and nature of the aforementioned 'socio-economic and cultural changes' (Hareven, 1995: 132) that have culminated in the emergence of old age as a life stage. It puts forward the view that old age as a life stage did not exist in preindustrial society; certain social, demographic, cultural and economic changes that occurred as result of industrialisation were highly influential in its construction as a life stage. In preindustrial society, communities were self-sufficient and older people were still land and property owners, everyone worked for most of their lifetime and there was far less of a distinction between those in their middle years and those in their later years. Families were also large and individual members were closely engaged with each other. Thus, older people were afforded considerable economic, social and familial power. However, during industrialisation, the move from the land to cities for work meant that older people lost the status previously derived from their work, land and property. There was also a reduction in family size and these smaller families were likely to live in the cities. Consequently, older people became socially and economically segregated. Life course explanations maintain that it was this constellation of changes that gradually led to their differentiation from other age groups and created a recognised formal phase of life for older people in society that was not solely related to biological ageing (Cohen, 1987; Hareven, 1995; Hockey and James, 2003; Hunt, 2005).

As indicated, these changes also impacted negatively on the lives and experiences of older people. According to the life course perspective, other social and cultural changes occurred that had further adverse implications for this group in society. These included the proliferation of negative stereotypes about older people, the growth in the literature on gerontology that highlighted the psychological and social problems of old age and the establishment of mandatory retirement and its concomitant association with dependency on social security (Hareven, 1995). Although this account portrays old age as being denigrated and associated with economic and social dependence, segregation and low status, recent work within the life course perspective argues that further 'socio-economic and cultural changes' have led to the dissipation of some of these features of old age. These include the raising of retirement age, the increase in workforce participation rates of older people, changing patterns of marriage and cohabitation and the increasing choice of lifestyles available to older people (Hunt, 2005; Vincent, 2006).

Other approaches within the life course perspective place particular emphasis on the role of the individual and the interplay between private lives and public events. One such approach can be found in work done by Holstein and Gubrium (2000). Their view is that within the constraints of social, cultural and historical circumstances individuals continuously construct their own life course; they argue that we are the 'everyday authors of our own lives' within 'circumstantial constraints' (Holstein and Gubrium, 2000: 182). However, these are not the only constraints on individuals' choice and autonomy in each life stage. Holstein and Gubrium argue that there are other constraints that result from interconnections between life stages and the way in which the character of a previous stage may influence future alternatives and patterns in the life course. The assimilation of these interconnections into Holstein and Gubrium's approach reflects the focus on the lack of clear-cut distinctions between stages in the life course perspective more generally, referred to above. The evidence about the persistence of inequalities from one life stage to another supports their arguments about the continuities that exist between the life stages (Arber and Ginn, 1995). For instance, studies on ageing have established that 'inequality in later life is related to employment status and socio-economic groups prior to retirement' (ibid.: 35).

The life course perspective in general has been accused of being 'vague at the theoretical level' (ibid.: 28) and not contributing to sociological theory. The justifications put forward for these accusations are that whilst material influences on the transitions in social life are highlighted, their sociological significance (such as their relative power) is not addressed. Nonetheless, despite these criticisms, the life course perspective has been praised for the way in which it acknowledges both collective experiences and the diversity of experience. Moreover, it is now used across many different areas, one of the most significant being health inequalities across the life course (Dike van de Mheen et al., 1998; Graham, 2002; Marmot, 2010). In order to gain an understanding of the ways in which the life course perspective has been applied to the study of health, we will first examine the relationship between our health and well-being and the life course. It is to this that we now turn.

The Life Course and Health and Well-Being

ACTIVITY 1.1

Before you start to read through this section, make a note of your thoughts about the relationship between health and the life course. Compare your ideas with the conclusions that emerge from the discussions of the data presented below.

A variety of indicators, such as self-reported health, **acute** and **chronic** illness rates and the incidence of mental illness, have been used to analyse the nature of the relationship between health and well-being and the life course (Larkin, 2011a). As demonstrated below, the results vary according to the indicators used and this relationship is far from straightforward.

Self-Reported Health

Table 1.1 shows that the percentage of both males and females in the population reporting 'good' general health declines across the life course as age increases. In addition, those reporting 'not good' health increases with advancing years, with the

Table 1.1 Self-reported health in Great Britain, by age and sex, 2006 (%)

Males	Good	Fairly good	Not good
0–15	85	12	3
16–24	83	14	3
25–44	74	20	6
45–64	58	28	14
65–74	44	36	19
75 and over	33	43	24
All ages	68	23	9
Females			
0–15	87	11	2
16–24	78	18	3
25–44	70	21	8
45–64	59	26	15
65–74	43	38	19
75 and over	33	39	28
All ages	66	23	11

Source: Office for National Statistics (2008: 25).

most significant increase being for those aged 75 and over. Therefore, Table 1.1 indicates that people *report* that their level of health progressively deteriorates as their chronological age increases.

However, analysis of the data on the incidence of acute, chronic and mental illness[1] show different patterns in the relationship between our health and our life course.

Acute Illness

Table 1.2 indicates that for both males and females, **acute illness** tends to decrease between the ages of 5 and 15 and then increase from 16 onwards, with the sharpest increases occurring after the age of 45.

Table 1.2   Acute illness: average number of restricted activity days per person per year, by sex and age, 2003–07

Males	2003	2004	2005	2006	2007
0–4	16	12	13	9	10
5–15	11	13	11	10	8
16–44	18	17	16	16	17
45–64	36	36	35	35	29
65–74	47	45	40	41	40
75 and over	56	59	54	56	45
Females					
0–4	14	16	11	10	10
5–15	11	8	8	11	7
16–44	22	22	24	21	21
45–64	42	41	37	40	37
65–74	57	52	57	55	43
75 and over	70	76	70	70	59

Source: Larkin (2011a: 85) based on original Office for National Statistics sources (2005, 2006, 2007, 2008, 2009a).

Chronic Illness

Two categories for **chronic illness** were used in the sources of data drawn on for this chapter. One was 'chronic longstanding illness', which refers to longstanding illness or disability. The other was 'chronic limiting longstanding illness', which is used for longstanding illness or disability that limits an individual's activity. Tables 1.3 and 1.4

---

[1]Tables 1.2 to 1.4 have been compiled using data from a number of General Household Surveys with the aim of showing trends over a minimum of five years. The range calendar of years and the age cohorts included within each table depended on the availability of comparable data.

show that increasing age brings with it a greater incidence of chronic illness for males and females, be it chronic longstanding illness or chronic limiting longstanding illness and disability, particularly amongst those who are over 65.

Table 1.3   Percentage reporting chronic longstanding illness, 2003–07

Males	2003	2004	2005	2006	2007
0–15	17	18	17	16	15
16–44	20	20	22	21	20
45–64	41	43	44	45	43
65+	62	60	61	66	62
Females					
0–15	15	14	14	14	13
16–44	22	32	24	23	22
45–64	41	62	43	44	41
65+	66	50	61	67	60

Source: Larkin (2011a: 86) based on original Office for National Statistics sources (2005, 2006, 2007, 2008, 2009a).

Table 1.4   Percentage reporting chronic limiting longstanding illness, 2003–07

Males	2003	2004	2005	2006	2007
0–15	6	7	7	6	5
16–44	10	10	11	10	11
45–64	24	26	26	23	25
65+	39	37	39	41	41
Females					
0–15	6	6	6	5	5
16–44	11	12	13	12	12
45–64	25	24	26	27	25
65+	41	40	43	45	42

Source: Larkin (2011a: 86) based on original Office for National Statistics sources (2005, 2006, 2007, 2008, 2009a).

Mental illness

The incidence of the different types of mental illnesses across the life course varies considerably. For instance, prevalence rates for depression below the age of 35 are lower than those for people aged between 35 and 59. Rates then fall noticeably for people aged 65 and over. In contrast, with the exception of those aged 45–54 who have substantially higher rates than other groups, anxiety disorder rates are relatively similar across all age groups whilst the prevalence of personality disorders increases steadily over the life course. Moreover, ascertaining the incidence of mental illness in general is problematic because of under-reporting, the accuracy of diagnostic tools and significant gender differences for some mental health problems such as eating disorders (McCrone et al., 2008). Hence, establishing the relationship between the incidence of mental health problems and age is challenging. However, there have been some attempts, one of the most recent being the English Longitudinal Study of Ageing (Department for Work and Pensions (DWP), 2009). This used a scoring system for mental health and well-being based on zero to four; those scoring zero were considered to be free of any form of mental illness and those who scored four or more were regarded as having some form of mental health problem. The average scores across the life course for males and females are presented in Table 1.5. The study found that those in the 65 to 79 age range have the least risk of mental ill health of any age group and overall those who are 80 plus have the worst mental health. This broadly U-shaped patterning in the overall incidence of mental health problems is supported by other research that has shown that mental distress is high in childhood, adolescence, young adulthood and very old age (Rogers and Pilgrim, 2003; Pilgrim, 2007; Allen, 2008).

Table 1.5 Average mental health scores in England, by age and sex (%)

Age range	Women (%)				Men (%)			
	16–49	50–64	65–79	80–plus	16–49	50–64	65–79	80–plus
Score 0	60	64	68	56	69	68	71	56
Score 1–3	25	20	21	29	21	20	20	26
Score 4+	15	16	10	15	10	12	9	18

Source: McCormick et al. (2009:16).

The Life Course Perspective on Health and Well-Being

The different indicators will be referred to again in several of the chapters of this book as they not only highlight some significant variations in health and well-being across the life course but also the complexity of the relationship between our health and well-being and our life course. For instance, acute illness and mental illness rates tend to be higher in the younger age groups and then decline before increasing. Those reporting that their level of health is 'not good' increases as their chronological age increases. Similarly, the incidence of chronic illness increases with age. However, these indicators do clearly demonstrate that health and well-being declines from around middle age and the worst health is experienced by those who are over 65, but particularly those over 75. Whilst many explanations have been developed to account for the variations in health and well-being across the life course, the way that there is a general decline in health and well-being from midlife onwards has received much theoretical attention. This is mainly because of the growing body of evidence that many risk factors for poorer health 'are rooted in people's experiences in the early years and that individuals exposed to severe adversity during their early years are at an increased risk of developing negative outcomes in later life' (Borgonovi, 2010: 1928). Such evidence is clearly aligned to arguments in the life course perspective and has stimulated the development of a life course approach to health (O'Donnell, 2005; Field and Taylor, 2007). It is this multidisciplinary approach – which is known as the life course perspective on health and well-being – that has contributed most to understandings of the patterning of health and illness over the whole life course. This section will discuss the life course perspective on health and well-being and then look at the many different areas in the study of health to which this perspective has been applied.

The Life Course Perspective on Health and Well-Being

The life course perspective on health and well-being starts from the premise that poorer health outcomes accumulate as we progress through each life stage. It argues that from conception, through to infancy, childhood, adolescence, adulthood and old age we are exposed to various risk factors. The health outcomes of these risks are shaped 'independently, cumulatively and interactively' (Kuh and Hardy, 2002: 5) by various environmental, psychological, social, historical and biological factors. In addition, this perspective recognises that positive experiences over the life course can offset exposure to negative events and risk factors (Kuh and Ben-Shlomo, 2005; Borgonovi, 2010).

There are many different models within the life course perspective on health and well-being. Some of those working within this approach argue that the health of a person involves the interaction between a biographical element and an historical element and have developed the concepts of 'biographical time' and 'historical time'. The former relates to how features of someone's personal biography, such as employment undertaken and personality influence their physical and mental health during their life course. For instance, employment based mainly around manual labour can lead to osteoarthritis from middle age onwards (Kubzansky et al., 2009). In relation to personality, studies have shown how specific childhood personality attributes, such as conscientiousness, ability to concentrate, distress proneness and behavioural inhibition influence adult health (Friedman et al., 1993; Sanders et al., 2002; Kubzansky et al., 2009). With reference to personal biographies and mental health specifically, psychological theories have long emphasised how experiences in childhood influence the incidence of mental health problems throughout the life course. Family environment has received much attention in these theories. Although there is an interaction with social class position, children who are subject to neglect and/or abuse are significantly more likely to be distressed or dysfunctional and experience increased rates of mental health problems as they progress through their adult lives (Pilgrim, 2007).

The concept of 'historical time' within this approach refers to the particular social and economic events that occur in the course of a person's life. These range from changing attitudes to health and sexuality through to economic recessions, political unrest and wars. It provides an understanding of how people's health and well-being is influenced by the particular generation or age cohort to which they belong. An example often cited to illustrate this point is the way that prior to the 1960s the serious threat to health posed by smoking was not recognised. The lack of knowledge about the dangers of smoking meant that preceding age cohorts had an increased vulnerability to the associated health risks. Studies into the other types of 'historical time' have shown how, for instance, those who experienced radical social changes in their youth see life as meaningful and want to stay physically and mentally active for as long as possible as they age. In addition, those who lived through the privations of the Second World War have been found to be better at self-denial and more able to cope with life's problems in adulthood (Vincent, 2006; Gunnarsson, 2009).

As mentioned above, in this approach to the life course perspective on health and well-being, 'biographical time' and 'historical time' are seen as relating to each other. This is because both negative and positive experiences in 'historical' time can influence 'biographical' time and vice versa. Moreover, the human body 'stores' the effects of the interactions between the beneficial and damaging experiences of 'biographical' and 'historical' time throughout the life course. Any damage accumulates and, if there is not an adequate balance between negative and positive experiences, health problems occur as we progress through our lives (Bury, 2000). These arguments are illustrated in the case study below.

David's Story

David had been happily married to Sue for ten years. He had worked as an Environmental Health Office since leaving university and really enjoyed his job as well as the contact with the public that it entailed. Sue was a music teacher and had reduced her work hours when their son was born four years earlier so that she could look after him. During the cuts in public spending in 2011, David was made redundant and was unable to find further employment. The financial and emotional strain of his unemployment took its toll on his marriage and he and Sue separated. According to the life course approach, the combined effects of damaging events in David's 'biographical' and 'historical' time will have negative impacts on his health in later life. However, his previous more positive experiences of marriage and employment in his 'biographical' time may well counteract some of these negative effects.

Others working within the life course perspective have adopted an **epidemiological** approach to health and well-being. This means that their focus is on the development of *disease* across the life course and they emphasise that it is the *timing* of exposure to events that determines their eventual impact on our health (Kuh and Ben-Shlomo, 2005; Lynch and Davey Smith, 2005). This literature refers to 'critical periods' or 'sensitive periods' in life during which exposure to particular events or risks has 'lasting or lifelong effects on the structure or function of organs, tissues and body systems which are not modified in any dramatic way by later experience' (Ben-Shlomo and Kuh, 2002: 285). Much of the work using an epidemiological approach to health and well-being has concentrated on prenatal and early life exposure to risks and their implications for health and well-being across the life course.

ACTIVITY 1.2

Which of the above points are illustrated in the following excerpt from Hilary Graham's (2009) work on health inequalities? There are some ideas to help you at the end of the chapter:

Fetuses, infants, children and adolescents pass through many critical and sensitive periods as they develop to maturity, particularly between conception and early childhood. This makes not only pregnancy but also childhood and adolescence, particularly in the early years, an unparalleled time during which external influences, both good and bad, can influence an individual's health and well-being across their whole life. Of particular importance is the health and circumstances of mothers, which links to their children's health through biological, behavioural and social mechanisms. (Graham, 2009: 26)

Contributions of the Life Course Perspective on Health and Well-Being

The models outlined above usefully identify different factors that affect our health and well-being across the life course. However, disentangling, let alone researching, all of the processes that purportedly affect our health and well-being throughout our lives is highly problematic. Hence, the life course perspective on health and well-being raises 'formidable methodological challenges' (Graham, 2007: 145). Nonetheless, it is credited with having led to the recognition of the development of disease over the whole life course in healthcare. This simultaneously led to the acknowledgement that the whole person within the ongoing context of their life in its entirety needs to be taken into consideration when addressing health issues. It has also inspired a raft of preventative policies aimed at preventing the development of health problems from the very beginning of life (Lynch et al., 1997; Bradshaw et al., 2006; Department of Health, 2010b). At a European level, the emphasis has recently been on ensuring that healthy ageing should start in childhood and take a lifelong perspective. Policies have focused on promoting healthy diets, physical activities, social relations and meaningful activities necessary for ageing healthily throughout a person's life (Stegeman et al., 2012). Consequently, the life course perspective on health and well-being has played a significant role in the swing from curative to preventative medicine in that it is central to the contemporary **public health** movement. This aims at improving lives by reducing the incidence of ill health and diseases at population and community level, rather than at an individual level. Examples of health issues addressed within public health are **obesity**, heart disease and mental illness. The focus of public health intervention in general is the prevention of health problems and identifying illness at a stage where treatment is more likely to be effective. A key element in its recent strategies is the use of a life course approach to track the causes, progression and pattern of physical and mental health problems in order to identify the most effective ways to prevent them from developing at different life stages (Orme et al., 2007; Department of Heath, 2009b, 2010b; Royal College of Psychiatrists, 2010). Furthermore, an increasing range of documents in other policy areas now adopt a life course approach to health and well-being. These include those aimed at tackling health inequalities, such as the *Marmot Review* (Marmot, 2010). This states that 'a life course perspective' is 'central to the Review' and that 'disadvantage starts before birth and accumulates throughout life'. Figure 1.1, which is used in the Review itself, illustrates this point and supports its contention that 'action to reduce health inequalities must start before birth and be followed through the life of the child'. The Review goes on to argue that it is only by doing this that 'the close links between early disadvantage and poor outcomes throughout life be broken' (ibid.: 14). Recent reforms to the social care system also reflect this approach (Department of Heath, 2010a).

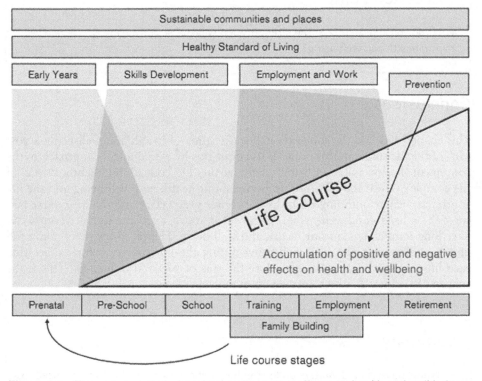

Figure 1.1   The accumulation of positive and negative effects on health and well-being across the life course

Source: Marmot (2010: 20).

There are many other areas of study where the life course perspective on health and well-being is influential. As its insights have led to an appreciation of the point that the true impact of inequality on individuals' health requires a consideration of the whole of their lives, it has acted as a catalyst for new research in the study of social inequalities in health. Consequently, a life course perspective is being increasingly used in developing the 'social inequalities in health' debate. One of its strengths in this area is that it integrates individual life trajectories with evolving social structures (Davey Smith et al., 2000). Particular social inequalities have recently received more attention than others, one of these being socioeconomic influences. The term 'life course socioeconomic status' has been used to refer to an individual's journey from the socioeconomic environment of their birth family (natal family) to adulthood. Studies have investigated how this journey affects health and show that those who experience the most exposure to poorer circumstances in their lives have poorer health (Graham, 2007). In addition, this perspective has been applied to the study of ageing, disability, mental illness and injury prevention (Kuh and Ben-Shlomo, 2005; Blanchflower and Oswald, 2008; Friedli, 2009; Priestly, 2010; Hosking et al., 2011).

Discussion Point

What do you consider to be the strengths and weaknesses of the life course perspective on health and well-being?

Conclusions

This chapter has laid the foundations for the study of health and well-being across each of the life stages in this book. It has done this by explaining its approach to the concept of 'health and well-being', defining the 'life course', highlighting some of the complexities of the relationship between our health and well-being and the life course, as well as outlining both the life course perspective and the life course perspective on health and well-being. As indicated above, exposure to risk *in utero* can have long-term effects on our health and well-being. Hence, in order to gain a full understanding of health and well-being during the life course, before addressing each life stage, it is essential to explore the role of prenatal influences. This is the subject of Chapter 2, to which we now turn.

Summary

- Whilst there is no definitive understanding of 'health and well-being', it is used to convey our feelings about ourselves as human beings, our lives and our relationships as an important component of our physical and mental health

- The growing recognition since the 1980s that our lives are not divided into well-defined and sequential stages has meant that the concept of the 'life course' has gradually replaced that of the 'life cycle' within academic disciplines outside of medicine
- Theoretical perspectives have adopted the concept of the 'life course', the life course perspective itself being the most widely recognised. This emphasises the fluidity of the stages in our life
- The relationship between health and well-being and the life course is complex
- The development of the multidisciplinary life course perspective on health and well-being has contributed significantly to understandings about the nature of this relationship
- There are many different models within the life course perspective on health and well-being but they all start from the premise that poorer health outcomes accumulate as we progress through each life stage
- The life course perspective on health and well-being has played a significant role in the swing from curative to preventative medicine in that it is central to the contemporary public health movement and has influenced many other areas of study

Further Study

For a more in-depth study of the concept of the 'life course' and the life course perspective in general, see S. Hunt *The Life Course: A Sociological Introduction* (Basingstoke: Palgrave Macmillan, 2005); and J. Hockey and A. James *Social Identities across the Life Course* (Basingstoke: Palgrave Macmillan, 2003). If you want to increase your understanding of the life course perspective in relation to health and well-being, it will be useful to look at work by Diana Kuh, Yoav Ben-Shlomo, George Davey-Smith and John Lynch, all of whom have published extensively in this area.

Activity Comments

The extract illustrates a more epidemiological approach to health and well-being across the life course. This is because of its emphasis on the timing of exposure to risk. In line with the life course perspective on health and well-being in general, Hilary Graham (2009) argues that there are favourable and unfavourable influences on our health and well-being. However, she does not explain how these interact.

2

Beginnings: Prenatal Health

Introduction

As mentioned in the Introduction, this book aims to provide you with a comprehensive account of health and well-being across the whole lifespan from a life course perspective. Central to this is the examination of the evidence about the role of prenatal influences from conception to birth on health and well-being at various life stages. Investigations into these influences can be traced back to the classic study of women who were pregnant during the 'Dutch Hunger Winter'. This was a famine in the occupied northern part of the Netherlands during the winter of 1944–45 and was caused by a combination of factors. These were the restrictions imposed by the German administration on food imports to the western Netherlands, an unusually early and harsh winter that severely impeded food transportation and the fact that much agricultural land was ruined by the retreating German army.

The starvation caused by the famine resulted in the deaths of a total of 18,000 people. Many studies of the effects of famine on human health have taken place using data from the 'Dutch Hunger Winter'. The study of women who were pregnant during this famine found that the conditions to which they were exposed had adverse effects on the children *in utero* in that they gave birth to smaller children whose cognitive development was more likely to be impaired than that of other children. Furthermore, when these children grew up and had children of their own, their children were also smaller than average and experienced more problems with their cognitive development (Stein et al., 1975). These findings have subsequently been endorsed at national and international levels and this study was the catalyst for further research into the prenatal origins of health and ill health (Ben-Shlomo and Kuh, 2002). Indeed, a number of recent studies investigating the long-term effects of fetal exposure to the 1918–19 influenza pandemic have been carried out internationally. This was the most lethal influenza pandemic in recent human history; it claimed at least 20 million lives worldwide, and more than 2.6 million of these deaths were in Europe alone. These studies have found that exposure *in utero* to the pandemic led to an increased probability of stroke, diabetes, kidney disorders, disability, poor self-reported health, difficulties with hearing, talking, walking and lifting, cardiovascular disease between the ages of 60 and 82, poorer educational attainment as well as lower income, lower socioeconomic status and lower chances of marriage. Some of these outcomes, such as poorer educational attainment, have been found to be typically larger for males than for females (Neelsen and Stratmann, 2012). Another outcome of the 'Dutch Hunger Winter' findings is that research in this area now includes preconceptual influences on health and ill health. This chapter therefore explores the main findings to date about pre-pregnancy and prenatal risks to health and their implications for health and well-being across the life course.

In the Beginning ... Pre-pregnancy Health

What does the following extract tell you about pre-pregnancy weight and fetal growth? The implications of the findings presented are discussed below:

> Each additional kg of pre-pregnancy weight increases gestational age-adjusted birthweight by approximately 10 g. Thus infants of women with a pre-pregnancy weight of 75 kg have a birthweight that is about 100 g greater than that of infants born to women with a pre-pregnancy weight of 65 kg (assuming the same height and gestational duration). Pre-pregnancy weight below 50 kg increases the risk for a small-for-gestational infancy by about 80 per cent. (Joseph and Kramer, 2005: 400)

ACTIVITY 2.1

There is now a wealth of literature on the influence of pre-pregnancy health on fetal development (Centre for Maternal and Child Enquiries (CMACE), 2007a). As the quotation in Activity 2.1 shows, there is evidence of a strong relationship between maternal pre-pregnancy weight and fetal growth. Such findings have recently been extended to include the relationship between pre-pregnancy obesity and early child-hood health; maternal pre-pregnancy obesity has been found to be associated with the diagnosis of asthma in offspring at the age of 3 years (Reichman and Nepomnyaschy, 2008). However, studies have also shown that it is not just whether a woman is the correct weight before she conceives that is important; in order to maximise her chances of conceiving a healthy fetus, she also needs to optimise her nutrition, avoid alcohol, take a folic acid supplement, cease smoking and avoid exposure to hazardous substances, pesticides, infections and radiation (CMACE, 2007b; Department of Health, 2009c; Petit et al., 2010). Although there have also been concerns about the role of paternal preconceptual health, apart from the rela-tionship between good parental health and fertility, the evidence to date shows that such concerns are unfounded. For instance, parental exposure to radiation does not increase risk of ill health among children subsequently conceived (Burt et al., 2004).

Known Risks *in Utero*

As we saw in Chapter 1, whilst other factors may be influential in later life, epide-miologists maintain that exposure to certain risks *in utero* can damage our anatomy and metabolic systems and have long-term effects on our health and well-being. Many prenatal risks have now been identified and new ones are emerging all the time as research in this area is developing rapidly. Examples of the most well-known risks are set out in this section, together with their implications for health and well-being across the life course. As you will see, several cause **poor fetal growth** and/or **preterm birth**, both of which have many implications for health in the longer term. Although the definitions of normal and abnormal fetal growth are controversial, when a fetus is small for its gestational age this is usually attributed to poor fetal growth. However, apart from poor growth, fetal size depends on many other fac-tors, such as maternal stature and ethnic origin (Perry and Lumey, 2005). Preterm birth refers to the birth of a baby at less than 37 weeks of gestation. Births at less than 32 weeks of gestation are known as very preterm births whilst those between 32 and 36 weeks of gestation are called moderately preterm births (Kramer et al., 2010). With reference to poor fetal growth, this is associated with a substantially higher risk of cardiovascular and metabolic diseases (such as diabetes), **hypertension** and obesity in adult life (Ben-Shlomo and Kuh, 2002; van Dijk et al., 2010). Preterm birth in general increases the risk of the baby having breathing and feeding problems and, in developed countries, is the main cause of infant mortality. Very preterm births can result in cerebral palsy and mental retardation. They have also been asso-ciated with an increased risk of asthma in young adulthood as well hypertension at this life stage (Crump et al., 2011a, 2011b).

Both poor fetal growth and preterm birth increase infants' vulnerability in the early weeks and months of their lives and place them at a greater risk of a wide variety of developmental problems that can have adverse effects on health and the quality of life throughout the life course (Davis and Sandman, 2006; Peebles et al., 2010; Vederhus et al., 2010). For example, poor fetal growth confers a risk of behavioural and emotional adversity related to **attention deficit hyperactivity disorder (ADHD)** in young adulthood (Strang-Karlsson et al., 2008). In addition, poor fetal growth and preterm birth result in **low birth weight** that refers to a baby who weighs less than 2500 grammes (5 lbs) at birth. Low birth weight has been directly associated with a range of adverse health outcomes, such as cardiovascular diseases, hypertension and diabetes, in both childhood and adulthood (Graham and Power, 2004; Graham, 2009). Positive associations between low birth weight and breast cancer in middle age have also been found (dos Santos Silva and de Stavola, 2002). Other more indirect health outcomes of low birth weight are starting to be identified as well. For instance, individuals who have a low birth weight have been found to be less likely to undertake physical activity in their leisure time in childhood and adulthood. As physical activity in leisure time is known to play an important role in the prevention of chronic disease, this obviously increases their risk of such diseases (Salonen et al., 2010). When each of the prenatal risks is discussed below, their role in poor fetal growth and preterm birth will be addressed, together with other threats to health and well-being that they pose.

Nutrition During Pregnancy

Poor maternal nutrition during fetal development is now seen as a key determinant of health in childhood and adult life. Hence there has been much emphasis on the role of maternal nutrition in fetal growth and development and pregnant women are routinely given advice on the quality of their diet, such as how much of each type of food to eat per day and which foods to eat in order to raise stores of vitamins, iron and calcium (Perry and Lumey, 2005; Department of Health, 2009c). This is accompanied by advice about the right amount of weight to gain and the association between obesity in pregnancy and having a baby with an abnormality or a stillbirth. Excessive weight gain in pregnancy also increases a mother's risk of long-term obesity (CMACE, 2010; Campbell et al., 2011). Nonetheless, there is evidence in developed countries that whilst improved diet increases a woman's own gestational weight, the effect on fetal growth is only modest (Joseph and Kramer, 2005). At the same time, knowledge about the risks associated with certain foods for fetal health has increased dramatically in recent years. An example is the link between toxoplasmosis and uncooked meat, fish, eggs, soft cheeses, unpasteurised milk and unwashed fruit and vegetables. Toxoplasmosis is a parasitic infection that many people will never know that they have had. Others will have mild flu-like symptoms and a few may experience a more long-term illness similar to glandular fever. The baby can be infected with toxoplasmosis while in the womb through transplacental transmission. Depending on which stage of pregnancy (see below for more details) this occurs, toxoplasmosis can lead to miscarriage, hydrocephalus (water on the brain), brain damage, epilepsy, deafness, blindness or growth problems (Robson and Waugh, 2008). In the light of this increased knowledge about such adverse effects of different food substances on fetal health, nutritional advice to pregnant women in developed countries now focuses more on what to avoid eating. This is illustrated in Box 2.1, which is an extract from the Department of Health's most recent book about pregnancy (Department of Health, 2009c). These books are regularly revised as more and more research is carried out into nutrition in pregnancy and new risks are identified (Department of Health, 2007; Larkin, 2011a). The information in Box 2.1 shows the depth and complexity of the dietary advice currently provided.

Box 2.1   Foods to avoid when pregnant

There are some foods that you should not eat when you are pregnant because they may make you ill or harm your baby.

You Should Avoid:

Some types of cheese. Don't eat mould-ripened soft cheese like Brie, Camembert and others with a similar rind. You should also avoid soft blue-veined cheese, like Danish blue. These are made with mould and they can contain listeria, a type of bacteria that can harm your unborn baby. Although listeriosis is a very rare infection, it is important to take special precautions during pregnancy because even the mild form of the illness in the mother can lead to miscarriage, stillbirth or severe illness in a newborn baby. You can eat hard cheeses such as cheddar and Parmesan and processed cheeses made from pasteurised milk such as cottage cheese, mozzarella and cheese spreads.

Paté. Avoid eating all types of paté, including vegetable patés, as they contain listeria.

Raw or partially cooked eggs. Make sure eggs are thoroughly cooked until the whites and yolks are solid. This prevents the risk of salmonella food poisoning. Avoid foods containing raw and undercooked eggs, such as homemade mayonnaise.

Raw or undercooked meat. Cook all meat and poultry thoroughly so that there is no trace of pink or blood. Take particular care with sausages and mincemeat. It is fine to eat steaks and other whole cuts of beef and lamb rare as long as the outside has been properly cooked or sealed.

Liver products. Don't eat liver or liver products, like liver paté or liver sausage, as they may contain a lot of vitamin A. Too much vitamin A could harm your baby.

Supplements containing vitamin A. Don't take high-dose multivitamin supplements containing vitamin A.

Some types of fish. Don't eat shark, marlin and swordfish and limit the amount of tuna you eat to no more than two steaks a week (about of 140 g cooked or 170 g raw each) or four cans a week (about 140 g when drained). These types of fish contain high levels of mercury which can damage your baby's developing nervous system.

Don't eat more than two portions of oily fish per week. Oily fish includes fresh tuna (but not canned tuna), salmon, mackerel, sardines and trout.

Raw shellfish. Eat cooked rather than raw shellfish as they can contain harmful bacteria and viruses that can cause food poisoning.

Peanuts. If you would like to eat peanuts or foods containing peanuts (such as peanut butter) during pregnancy, you can choose to do so as part of a healthy balanced diet, unless you are allergic to them or your health professional advises you not to. You may have heard that some women have, in the past, chosen not to eat peanuts when they are pregnant. This is because the government previously advised women that they may wish to avoid eating peanuts during pregnancy if there was a history of allergy in their child's immediate family (such as asthma, eczema, hayfever, food allergy or other types of allergy). But this advice has now been changed because the latest research has shown that there is no clear evidence to say if eating or not eating peanuts during pregnancy affects the chances of your baby developing a peanut allergy.

Unpasteurised milk. Drink only pasteurised or UHT milk which has been pasteurised. If only raw or green-top milk is available, boil it first. Don't drink unpasteurised goats' or sheep's milk or eat certain food that is made out of them, e.g. soft goat's cheese. (Department of Health, 2009c)

ACTIVITY 2.2

As we have seen, there is a range of nutritional risk factors in utero which can have lasting effects on health during the life course. Read through the following extract about the role of nutrition in fetal growth and see which points were discussed above. Does this extract give you any additional insights into nutrition in pregnancy?

Fetal growth depends on the mother's nutritional status before conception, her diet during pregnancy, and interactions between these factors and aspects of the mother's metabolism and physiology such as glucose tolerance and **blood pressure**. In communities that provide adequate nutrition to sustain optimal growth in childhood and adolescence, dietary intake during pregnancy probably accounts for a relatively small amount of variation in fetal growth. Aspects of the mother's metabolism and physiology that determine the maternal uterine milieu are influenced by a range of genetic and environmental factors that are potentially important confounders in studies of association between fetal growth and adult disease. (Perry and Lumey, 2005: 363)

Maternal Alcohol Consumption

Whereas previously the occasional drink (one or two units once or twice a week) was considered safe for a pregnant woman, government advice now states that pregnant women should avoid alcohol altogether. This is because alcohol intake in pregnancy is associated with elevated risk of spontaneous preterm delivery and fetal abnormalities that have lifelong effects. These abnormalities include a range of physical and neurodevelopmental problems as well as **Fetal Alcohol Spectrum Disorders (FASD)**. The latter occur because of the way in which alcohol damages fetal brain development and the central nervous system. This damage can cause 'distinctive facial deformities, physical and emotional developmental problems, memory and attention deficits and a variety of cognitive and behavioural problems' (British Medical Association Board of Science, 2007: 2). These impairments are usually irreversible and persist into adulthood, often resulting in an inability to live independently in adulthood. Unfortunately, approximately one in twenty-five women **binge drink** during pregnancy and this increases the aforementioned risks (Aliyu et al., 2010; Peadon et al., 2010; Peebles et al., 2010; Freunscht and Feldmann, 2011).

Maternal Mental Health

Research into the effects of maternal mental health during pregnancy on the fetus has focused mainly on prenatal stress and depression. Taking maternal prenatal stress first, the fact that this can significantly impair fetal growth and shorten gestation leading to reduced infant birth weight is now well-established (Wadhwa et al., 1993, 2001; Davis and Sandman, 2006; Brown et al., 2011). In addition to the more general health implications of these outcomes, some studies have also identified specific negative and long-lasting consequences of high maternal anxiety levels during pregnancy for child development. For instance, antenatal maternal anxiety has been associated with lower mental developmental scores at the age of two years (Brouwers et al., 2001), attention deficit hyperactivity disorder (ADHD) symptoms as well as **externalising behaviour problems**, and anxiety in 8- and 9-year-olds (Van den Bergh et al., 2004). Other studies have found that cortisol levels in children and adolescents may be disturbed by the lasting effects that prenatal anxiety has on hypothalamic-pituitary-adrenal (HPA) axis functioning, thereby increasing their vulnerability to impaired learning and **psychopathology** (O'Connor et al., 2005; Davis and Sandman, 2006). Exposure to maternal stress during intrauterine life may also increase the risk in young adulthood of a range of negative physical and mental health outcomes, such as glucose-insulin, lipid metabolic dysfunction, immune dysfunction, hypothalamic-pituitary-adrenal endocrine dysregulation and cognitive (working memory) dysfunction (Entringer et al., 2008, 2010). Recent evidence also suggests that maternal stress during fetal development predisposes individuals to cardiovascular disease in both childhood and adult life (van Dijk et al., 2010).

With reference to maternal antenatal depression, this has been found to alter the development of stress-related biological systems in the fetus and increase the risk of birth complications and stillbirths. Other adverse outcomes are sleep problems in newborn babies that can persist through to 30 months, elevations in externalising behaviour problems in 8-year-olds and increased vulnerability to depression and abnormalities of their **neuroendocrine systems** in later life (Goodman and Rous, 2010; Department of Health, 2011c).

However, factors such as genetic inheritance may also play a role in some of these adverse health, developmental and adjustment outcomes. For instance, a study conducted by Rice et al. (2010) about exposure to prenatal stress found that ADHD in offspring was attributable to inherited factors. Other influences are good levels of social support and moderate income, both of which have been found to attenuate maternal prenatal stress (Ruckstuhl et al., 2010). Moreover, the *level* of prenatal stress has been shown to be an important influence in that mild to moderate levels of psychological distress may enhance fetal maturation in healthy populations (DiPietro et al., 2006).

Maternal Smoking

Smoking in pregnancy harms the developing fetus in many ways, for instance it restricts its essential oxygen. Evidence of these harmful effects has emerged from studies that have compared babies born to women who smoke in pregnancy and those born to women who do not smoke whilst pregnant; the former are more likely to be preterm (and experience all of the accompanying health problems as described above) and are more prone to infection. In their first year of life, the incidence of bronchitis, pneumonia and cot death is higher amongst the babies of women who smoke in pregnancy. They also have higher **mortality rates,** and have an increased risk of respiratory disease and asthma in childhood, psychiatric problems in young adulthood as well as heart attacks and strokes in midlife. Secondhand smoke has similar effects. Therefore, living with a partner who smokes and/or has regular exposure to smoke-filled environments during pregnancy can be as threatening to health and well-being across the life course as maternal prenatal smoking (Department of Health, 2009c; Perry and Lumey, 2005).

Medication in Pregnancy

Whilst pregnant women are encouraged as a matter of course to seek medical advice before taking any form of medication, for some women with chronic conditions, such as diabetes and epilepsy, pregnancy without medication is not an option for them and for the health of their baby. Using diabetes as an example, the maternal health risks of uncontrolled **Type 1** or **Type 2 diabetes** in pregnancy include heart disease, blindness and renal failure and there is a greater risk of the baby having a congenital malformation than if it is controlled (CMACE, 2007b). With reference to the use of medication to treat epilepsy, some antiepileptic drugs 'are associated with twofold to threefold increase in rates of major congenital malformations compared with the general population' (Nulman, 2010: 341). Rigorous assessment of the reproductive safety of all medication and judicious counselling is therefore required to produce the most favourable outcomes for maternal and fetal health.

Pre-pregnancy and Prenatal Risks: Real Risks to Health and Well-Being?

The ways in which the above prenatal risks *can* threaten health and well-being during the life course was explained in the discussion of each one. Some of the epidemiological literature on health and well-being across the life course adopts a deterministic approach in that such risks are seen as inevitably leading to trajectories of compromised health and well-being. This is illustrated in arguments put forward by those working within this approach that exposure to risks *in utero* can 'permanently alter anatomical structures and a variety of metabolic systems' (Ben-Shlomo and Kuh, 2002: 285), which in turn causes a variety of disorders both in childhood and in later life (ibid.; Lynch and Davey Smith, 2005). However, as indicated above in the exploration of maternal prenatal stress, other factors also play an important role in determining the outcomes of prenatal risks. Indeed, there is much evidence that exposure to risks *in utero* does not necessarily have damaging effects on a baby's health or on health and well-being in later life and several modifying factors have been identified.

Many studies have shown that the *timing* of exposure to risks *in utero* is important in determining their actual impact (see Chapter 1). These studies often use the concepts of 'critical periods' or 'sensitive periods' in fetal development and have focused on what are referred to as the **pregnancy trimesters**. Pregnancy is typically broken into three trimesters to describe the changes that take place. Each trimester is about three months: the first trimester is weeks 1 to 12; the second is weeks 13 to 27; and the third, weeks 28 to 42. Some of these studies have shown that exposure to risks in early pregnancy is more likely to have adverse effects on health than at other stages of pregnancy (Nulman, 2010; van Dijk et al., 2010; Neelsen and Stratmann 2012). Using toxoplasmosis as an example, there is a high risk of miscarriage if this infection is caught in early pregnancy and transmitted to the baby. Should the baby be infected during either the first or second trimester and the mother does not miscarry, he or she may be born with hydrocephalus (water on the brain), brain damage, epilepsy, deafness, blindness or growth problems. These developmental problems may be so severe that the pregnancy ends in a stillbirth. The problems are not so severe if toxoplasmosis is caught and transmitted to the baby in the third trimester of pregnancy. However, although it may appear that there is nothing obviously wrong at birth, health problems may develop, particularly with vision, later in life (Robson and Waugh, 2008). Other studies have shown that certain conditions are linked to exposure to risk factors *in utero* in later pregnancy. For instance, coronary heart disease in adult life has been linked to poor maternal nutrition in the second and third trimesters of pregnancy (Perry and Lumey, 2005).

Nonetheless, unborn babies vary in their susceptibility and some are more vulnerable at certain times and in certain ways than others. There is evidence that whilst some babies who seem to have incurred only slight risks before birth sadly suffer some degree of damage to their health and well-being, there are babies who have been exposed to several risks *in utero* who are born perfectly normal and healthy (Perry and Lumey, 2005). Although further research is required, some of this research has also indicated that male fetuses are more vulnerable *in utero* than female fetuses (van Dijk et al., 2010).

With reference to effects on health in later life, health problems linked to risks *in utero* may only develop if individuals experience exposure to other risks in their lives. An example is the way that obesity in childhood, adulthood or both increases the chances of developing coronary heart disease in adult life for those who have been exposed *in utero* to risks linked with this disease, such as poor maternal nutrition in the second and third trimesters of pregnancy (see above). Evidence about such modifiers has led to the conclusion that even if an individual has 'a biologically compromised system' because of exposure to risks *in utero*, this 'may only result in pathology with the subsequent addition of other physiological or metabolic stressors' (Davey Smith and Ebrahim, 2002: 286). This view that prenatal risks can be modified throughout the life course is supported by evidence that environmental and social factors influence health outcomes throughout the life course. For instance, children in lower socioeconomic groups are more likely to have emotional and behavioural problems, and both children and adults in lower socioeconomic groups are more likely to suffer from chronic diseases such as asthma and cardiovascular disease. Similarly, the higher incomes experienced by those in the higher socioeconomic groups and their more positive health behaviours can reduce the extent to which prenatal risks to health have an adverse affect on health and well-being throughout the life course (Graham, 2007, 2009).

Despite all of this evidence about the role of modifying factors, it is clear that the significance of fetal exposures should not be underestimated. Those who adopt a less deterministic approach to the epidemiology of health and well-being across the life course emphasise this point. This group acknowledges that the occurence of some disorders linked to exposure risks *in utero* can be reduced by factors that promote good health in later life and exposures to risks in later life do influence disease risk. It does argue, however, that it is fetal exposures that have the more *permanent* effects on our health and well-being (Ben-Shlomo and Kuh, 2002; Graham and Power, 2004).

Discussion Point

To what extent do you agree with those epidemiologists who adopt a more deterministic approach and see prenatal risks as inevitably leading to compromised health and well-being?

Reducing the Risks

As we have seen, there is much advice for women who either intend to conceive or are pregnant about reducing pre-pregnancy and prenatal risks. In addition, many healthcare interventions have been developed to minimise these risks. Examples include those that have addressed smoking cessation in pregnancy and reducing the risks of pregnancy for obese women (Koshy et al., 2010; Nagle et al., 2011). Although women can use the information available to reduce known pre-conceptual and prenatal risks, this is easier for some than for others; socioeconomic and interpersonal resources have been found to influence prenatal health behaviours, with women in higher socioeconomic groups and those with greater interpersonal resources exhibiting the most positive prenatal behaviours. Findings about class differences in prenatal health behaviour accords with those about class differences in health-related behaviour more generally. These show that those in the lower classes tend to take more risks in relation to their health (Larkin, 2011a). With reference to interpersonal resources, these are reduced in strained personal relationships (including those in which there is relationship conflict and physical abuse). Whilst this finding in itself is not unexpected, what is of greater consequence is that the stress subsequently experienced has been shown to be associated with poor prenatal health behaviour (Kimbro, 2008). Hence, the fact that some women do not adhere to the guidance given to them about their prenatal health behaviour may reflect external factors over which they have limited control.

Moreover, as demonstrated, some of the factors that increase vulnerability to prenatal risks *in utero* can be outside an individual's immediate control. The issue of maternal poverty has received particular attention. This is because research has shown that poorer mothers are more likely to give birth to smaller babies or deliver them preterm. In addition, the infant mortality rate is 17 per cent higher for the lowest two socioeconomic groups compared to the rest of the population (Graham and Power, 2004; Graham, 2009). Another influence is race; there are racial disparities in preterm birth and infant mortality rates (Kramer et al., 2010; Lu et al., 2010). Fetal growth can be adversely affected by a mother's nutritional levels during her own childhood and adolescence, as well as maternal and fetal genotypes (Perry and Lumey, 2005). Medical practice, such as assisted reproductive technology, interventions in pregnancy and the medical induction of preterm births may also impact negatively on fetal health and well-being during the life course (Kramer et al., 2010; VanderWeele et al., 2012). As demonstrated in Box 2.2, recent research has shown that boys conceived through IVF may experience infertility. New medical strategies used to prolong gestation when spontaneous preterm delivery is a risk or starts to occur have also become a matter of concern recently. These are based on the assumption that neonatal and therefore childhood outcomes are better the longer that gestation proceeds and delaying delivery is beneficial. However, there is evidence to suggest that some interventions that prolong pregnancy may have delayed detrimental effects. For instance, the administration of certain antibiotics (erythromycin and co-amoxiclav) during spontaneous preterm labour can increase the chances of a child having cerebral palsy (Peebles et al., 2010).

Box 2.2   The risks of IVF treatment

Test-Tube Babies May Inherit Fertility Problems

Doctors have uncovered the first evidence that fathers of test-tube babies may be passing on their infertility to their sons. A new study has found that boys conceived through IVF treatment involving a single sperm being directly injected into a female egg often inherit shorter fingers, a trait known to be associated with infertility. The result raises the prospect of a new and growing generation who may be less likely to have children of their own. Almost 1 in 50 British babies are conceived artificially and nearly half the couples having treatment go through a treatment procedure known as ICSI (intracytoplasmic sperm injection). The technique bypasses the normal competition where only the healthiest sperm cell is able to reach the female egg and fertilize it. Alastair Sutcliffe, a pediatrician at the Institute of Child Health in London, led the Anglo-German study which compared 211 six-year-olds conceived through ICSI with 195 naturally conceived children of the same age. The ICSI groups were similar heights to the naturally conceived group, but the boys had significantly shorter fingers. It is known that men with low sperm counts often have ring fingers the same length as their index finger, whereas fertile men are more likely to have a ring finger which is relatively longer than their index finger ... . 'This is the first study of this kind on these children,' Sutcliffe said. 'We don't yet know the implications of the findings because the children are very young, but we need to inform people (about the possible risks of the ICSI procedure)'. ... Finger length is known to be set within the first 14 weeks of pregnancy and is linked to testosterone exposure which is, in turn, governed by a specific group of genes ... . 'This (research) is telling us that we should only use ICSI when it is absolutely necessary,' said John Manning, an evolutionary biologist at Southampton University ... . 'We know the extraordinary depression and pain that childlessness can cause and we have a responsibility to ensure that the focus on the well-being of children born as result of these techniques is as high as it can be.' (Rogers, 2010)

Therefore the discussions in this section raise some important issues about reducing pre-pregnancy and prenatal risks. These are that even though information about ways of reducing these risks to health and well-being across the life course may be effectively disseminated, successful outcomes are contingent on many variables that are beyond control at an individual level. Moreover, the full range of these variables has yet to be identified, as evidenced by the fact that research is constantly uncovering further prenatal risks. A very recent study found that a mother's exposure to air pollution (such as pollution for the burning of fossil fuels for transport and heating, as well as energy production) when pregnant can impair a child's cognitive ability (Lovasi et al., 2010).

Discussion Point

What advice do you think that health professionals should give to pregnant women about securing the best outcomes in terms of health and well-being for their babies?

Conclusions

This chapter has explored the role of some of the known pre-pregnancy and prenatal risks on the unborn child and his or her health and well-being across the life course. This exploration showed how the effects of these can be modified both *in utero* and at other stages during our lives by a range of influences. Examples of these are genetic, social, environmental and technological factors, many of which we are unable to control as individuals. Thus, as well as focusing on advising women about preconceptual and prenatal risks in order to achieve the optimal outcomes for health and well-being, there needs to be more research into the wider influences on fetal health. Furthermore, policies need to continue to address those already identified and those that emerge as a result of future research.

The exploration of pre-pregnancy and prenatal risks included the debates about the extent to which fetal exposures can have permanent effects on our health and well-being. As we saw in Chapter 1, there are arguments put forward by those working within the life course approach to health and well-being that 'not only pregnancy but also childhood and adolescence' are 'an unparalleled time during which external influences, both good and bad, can influence an individual's health and well-being across their whole life' (Graham, 2009: 26). The next two chapters will examine the validity of these claims with respect to childhood and adolescence. We will start by looking at childhood in Chapter 3.

Summary

- There is now a substantial body of literature on the influence of pre-pregnancy health on fetal development and how women can maximise their chances of conceiving a healthy fetus
- The evidence that exposure to certain risks *in utero* can damage the fetus and have long-term effects on our health and well-being has increased considerably in recent

years, with new risks regularly being identified. Amongst the most well-known risks are maternal nutrition, stress, smoking, alcohol consumption and medication during pregnancy

- The extent to which prenatal risks do damage to a baby's health as well as health and well-being in later life has been the subject of much debate. Some adopt a deterministic approach. Others, whilst acknowledging the significance of the role of fetal exposures, argue that other factors can modify prenatal risks throughout the life course
- Even if women do adhere to advice they are given about reducing preconceptual and prenatal risks, some influential factors whilst a baby is *in utero* are beyond individual control. Examples of these factors are poverty, race, genetic inheritance and the possible effects of medical intervention in conception and pregnancy

Further Study

As mentioned, this is a dynamic area and new research findings are emerging all of the time. You will find the most up-to-date studies in journals such as *BMC Public Health*, The *British Medical Journal* and the *European Journal of Public Health*. For a more detailed discussion of fetal growth, see the chapters by I.J. Perry and L.H. Lumey and K.S. Joseph and M.S. Kramer in D. Kuh and Y. Ben-Shlomo (eds), *A Lifecourse Approach to Chronic Disease Epidemiology*, 2nd edn (Oxford: Oxford University Press, 2005).

There are numerous websites that offer advice on maximising a baby's prenatal health. Amongst the most informative are the National Childbirth Trust (www.nct.org.uk) and Patient UK (www.patient.co.uk/doctor/Pre-pregnancy-Counselling.htm). Articles by Yoav Ben-Shlomo, Diane Kuh and George Davey Smith are a very useful source if you want more information about work in this area from an epidemiological perspective.

3

Health and Well-Being in Childhood

Introduction

The concept of childhood is contestable; many point to the way that childhood varies historically, socially and culturally and argue that it is socially constructed. The complexity of such arguments is further compounded by the fact that 'childhood' can refer to a varying range of years in terms of cognitive, physical, social and emotional development (Beckett, 2009; Larkin, 2009). Whilst recognising these arguments as well as the sequential and critical nature of the developmental stages that take place in childhood, for the purposes of exploring health and well-being in childhood in this chapter we will focus on children from birth up to around the end of their first decade of life.

The data about health and well-being across the life course presented in Chapter 1 showed that although acute and chronic illness rates are higher in early childhood than in later childhood, these rates are lower during childhood in general than in other life stages. However, along with young adulthood and very old age, childhood is a time of higher rates of mental distress. The chapter will start by looking at the evidence about the health and well-being of this age group in more depth. In order to assess the claim that childhood is one of those 'unparalleled' times in life in terms of how 'external influences, both good and bad, can influence an individual's health and well-being across their whole life' (Graham, 2009: 26), the chapter will then address three key issues using a life course perspective. The first of these issues is the role of pre-pregnancy and prenatal influences on health and well-being in childhood. The second area of focus is the extensive literature about the risks that children can be exposed to and how these can affect their health and well-being during childhood as well as in other stages of their lives. The potential impact of other factors on these risks in determining their outcomes is the third main issue. The chapter will end with an overview of approaches adopted in policies aimed at addressing issues around children's health and well-being. Any distinctions between early and later childhood will be highlighted in the discussions.

Children's Health and Well-Being

Despite the fact that the comprehensiveness and validity of data on children's health have been criticised, some clear trends have emerged in recent years. Infant and childhood mortality rates (including accidental deaths) have decreased substantially over the past two decades. Although children still experience common childhood illnesses such as chickenpox, whooping cough, three-day-fever and croup, the overall health of children in the United Kingdom dramatically improved throughout the last century. This improvement has been attributed to the fact that contagious diseases (examples of which include measles, diptheria, polio and tuberculosis) have almost been eradicated and the continuing development of successful treatments for previously fatal diseases (Timimi, 2004; Beresford et al., 2005). In contrast, the prevalence of mental health disorders has increased; studies show that the most frequently occurring conditions are emotional, hyperactive and **conduct disorders** (Quilgars et al., 2005; McCrone et al., 2008; Graham, 2009). A conduct disorder that is currently of particular concern is the aggression (verbal and physical) used by children in parent–child relationships. This has increased in scale and intensity. Whilst it is recognised that physical and verbal aggression are part of normal child development, the evidence gathered indicates that many of the children who are displaying such aggression are not enjoying good mental health and well-being and may be at risk of developing complex emotional disorders (Parentline Plus, 2010). Indeed, studies of developed countries show that levels of child well-being in the United Kingdom compare very unfavourably with other developed countries, including substantially poorer ones (United Nations Children's Fund, 2007). Other new health issues amongst children have also been identified. Examples of these are the rises in chronic illnesses and obesity rates. With reference to chronic illnesses, the greatest relative rise in the prevalence of Type 1 diabetes and asthma has been amongst those under 16 years of age. Britain now has one of the highest prevalence rates for childhood asthma in the world; the increases have been highest in those in the lower socioeconomic groups and those of Asian origin (Beresford et al., 2005). There is also national and international concern about obesity rates in childhood; in the United Kingdom, almost a quarter of children are now **overweight** or obese by the time that they start primary school, and this figure rises to more than a third by the time they leave (Department of Health, 2009a). These figures are predicted to increase further but of greater concern is the fact that they do not reflect the true extent of the problem because studies indicate that overweight prevalence rates in children are often underestimated (Finch and Searle, 2005; *Foresight Report*, 2007; Scoltens et al., 2007).

Life Before Childhood

At the beginning of this book, we saw how the life course perspective has led to the recognition that poorer health outcomes are cumulative from conception through to old age. In Chapter 2, a range of pre-pregnancy and fetal exposures that can compromise health in childhood were discussed. These are summarised in Table 3.1. As explained previously, new findings about health and well-being across the life course are constantly emerging. Therefore, the summary presented is not a definitive list of all of the risks to health and well-being in childhood that can occur both before and during pregnancy. Rather, it aims to reflect those identified in Chapter 2 and to demonstrate their potential cumulative effects during childhood.

As we saw in Chapter 2, integral to an explanation of the influence of pre-pregnancy and fetal exposures in childhood is an appreciation of how they can be modified by a range of individual, environmental and social factors. These can have both positive and negative effects and are extremely hard to unravel. The discussion of maternal prenatal stress in Chapter 2 illustrated this point well; this showed how factors such as genetic inheritance, social support, income and level of stress may influence the health, developmental and adjustment outcomes of maternal prenatal stress. For example, good levels of social support and moderate income have been found to attenuate maternal prenatal stress. In addition, mild to moderate levels of psychological distress may have positive effects on fetal maturation. Despite the existence of such complicated interactions, the literature on pre-pregnancy and prenatal influences does contribute to our understanding of childhood health from a life course perspective. An examination of the risks to health and well-being that can occur during childhood itself is required in order to develop this understanding further and it is to these risks that we now turn.

Table 3.1 The role of pre-pregnancy and fetal exposures in childhood health and well-being

Pre-pregnancy influences	Outcomes in childhood
Maternal pre-pregnancy weight below 50 kg	Poor fetal growth that increases vulnerability in the early weeks and months of infants' lives and places them at greater risk of a wide variety of developmental problems. It can also lead to low birth weight. This can result in a range of adverse health outcomes in childhood, such as cardiovascular diseases, hypertension and diabetes
Maternal pre-pregnancy obesity	Associated with diagnosis of asthma at three years of age
Fetal exposures	
Low-quality maternal diet	Poor fetal growth and low birth weight that can result in cardiovascular diseases, hypertension and diabetes in childhood
Obesity in pregnancy	Increases risk of abnormality or a stillbirth
Risks associated with certain foods such as uncooked meat, fish, eggs	Hydrocephalus (water on the brain), brain damage, epilepsy, deafness, blindness and growth problems
Maternal alcohol consumption	Physical and neurodevelopmental problems as a result of fetal abnormalities. Examples of these problems are facial deformities, physical and emotional developmental problems, memory and attention deficits, as well as cognitive and behavioural problems
Prenatal stress	As this can lead to low birth weight, the risks of cardiovascular diseases, hypertension and diabetes are increased in childhood. Other outcomes in childhood are lower mental developmental scores at the age of two years, attention deficit hyperactivity disorder (ADHD) symptoms as well as externalising problems, and anxiety in 8- and 9-year-olds. Some studies have also found links with increased vulnerabilities to cardiovascular disease and impaired learning and psychopathology
Maternal antenatal depression	Increased risk of birth complications, stillbirths, sleep problems in newborn babies that can persist through to 30 months, and externalising behaviour problems in 8-year-olds
Smoking and regular exposure to smoke-filled environments in pregnancy	Preterm birth that in general increases the risk of a baby having breathing and feeding problems and, in developed countries, is the main cause of infant mortality. Very preterm births can result in cerebral palsy and mental retardation. In their first year of life, babies who are born preterm are also more prone to infections, respiratory disease (such as bronchitis and asthma), pneumonia and cot deaths, as well as higher mortality rates
Uncontrolled Type 1 or Type 2 diabetes	Congenital malformation

Risks to Health and Well-Being During Childhood

The emphasis in this section will be on the ways in which the risks to health and well-being that can occur during childhood can compromise health and well-being during childhood itself and threaten health and well-being at other stages in the life course. The discussions will include reference to contextual features where these have been identified in the existing body of research.

ACTIVITY 3.1

The grid set out below uses the same format as that in Table 3.1. As you read through the rest of this section, try to identify any risks that are likely to affect health and well-being at the next life stage – adolescence. Make a note of them on the grid. This activity is designed to help you develop your ability to interpret the findings about health and well-being at a particular life stage from a life course perspective.

Childhood risks	Outcomes for health and well-being in adolescence

Birth

Despite reductions in infant mortality rates and advances in obstetric care, being born is still an inherently dangerous and risky activity. The risks include injuries to the skeleton and fracture of the clavicle, head trauma and **perinatal asphyxia**. Such major birth trauma can contribute to increased neonatal **morbidity** and mortality as well as have a negative impact on health and well-being in later life. For instance, babies that experience perinatal asphyxia usually require treatment in a special care unit because they are weak and unresponsive. Perinatal asphyxia can also result in **encephalopathy** and multiple organ dysfunction, both of which can cause irreversible damage (Nabieva, 2007; Aiyama et al., 2009; Sauber-Schatz et al., 2010; Department of Health, 2011c). Other factors, such as the time of day at which a baby is born, can increase the risk associated with being born, too; babies born at night have been shown to have a 22 per cent higher risk of encephalopathy (Hopkins Tanne, 2010). Furthermore, there are less direct but nonetheless significant effects of serious birth trauma. These stem from the way in which a traumatic birth experience can lead to childbirth-related post-traumatic stress disorder in mothers.

Amongst the outcomes of such disorders is an inability to bond with the child that has long-term effects on a child's psychological health and cognitive development (Alcorn et al., 2010).

Breastfed or Not?

Whilst formula feeding has many health advantages, breastfeeding does result in considerable reductions in risks to health and well-being in infancy, childhood and throughout the life course. In addition, its beneficial effects generally increase with the length of breastfeeding. During infancy, these include a decrease in the incidence and severity of many infections in infancy, such as gastroenteritis and respiratory infections. Recent research about breastfeeding and outcomes in childhood have shown that it is associated with a lower risk of being overweight or obese, fewer behavioural problems and improved cognitive development and academic performance. It also reduces the risk of suffering from several illnesses in childhood. These include diabetes, leukaemia, asthma and eczema. With respect to adulthood, breastfeeding can provide protection from later adverse health outcomes, for example diabetes and coronary heart disease (Gillman, 2005; Martin et al., 2005; Walker, 2006). Being breastfed has also been found to lead to higher psychological well-being in women throughout the life course (Cable et al., 2011). However, such associations are controversial because of numerous confounding factors, such as the maternal and socioeconomic characteristics (Holme et al., 2010; Heikkilä et al., 2011; McCrory and Layte, 2011; McVeigh, 2011). Last but not least, the benefits of breastfeeding extend to mothers' longer-term health as well; it increases the likelihood that mothers use up body fat deposited during pregnancy and can reduce the likelihood of developing some forms of ovarian cancer and premenopausal breast cancer (Kelly and Watt, 2005; Dyson et al., 2007).

Maternal Depression

Postnatal depression affects approximately one in ten new mothers and has been linked with increased risk of infections in children up to the age of 4 years (Ban et al., 2010; Parentline Plus, 2010). As childhood infections have been shown to play a role in adult chronic diseases (for example, cardiovascular disease), maternal postnatal depression can therefore also have implications for morbidity in adulthood (Davey Smith and Lynch, 2005). Studies of mothers who suffer from postnatal depression have shown that their illness can result in them being unresponsive, critical and unpredictable as parents. The adoption of such negative parenting styles can impact on **mother–child attachment** that leads to cognitive and emotional developmental problems. There is evidence that such problems are not only associated with a child being 'almost 12 times more likely to have a statement for social needs for emotional, behavioural or learning problems at school' (Parentline Plus, 2010:

14), but also 'with a five-fold increased risk of later mental health problems' (Department of Health, 2011c: 10). Nonetheless, the potential for transactional processes, such as how a child's characteristics, age of the mother and poverty, contribute to the development and maintenance of depression in mothers' needs to be assessed before specific associations between postnatal depression and health and well-being can be made (Goodman and Rous, 2010; Department of Health, 2011c). Furthermore, as general maternal health as well as psychological well-being during the early years of raising children may be equally influential, this also needs to be taken into consideration (Mensah and Kiernan, 2011).

Childhood Illnesses

Specific associations between poor childhood health and increased morbidity in later life have been found for cancer, lung disease, arthritis, rheumatism and cardiovascular conditions (Blackwell et al., 2001; Kuh et al., 2005). In addition, studies have shown that some of the illnesses experienced by infants and children are likely to have 'long-term consequences for adult morbidity, disability and handicap' (Kuh et al., 2005: 379). Examples of these are the illnesses affecting their respiratory, circulatory, alimentary and urogenital systems, as well as chronic illnesses such as psoriasis, epilepsy and diabetes. Conditions, such as **congenital heart defects** (**CHD**), can also lead to communication and social impairment (Brandlistuen et al., 2011). Other childhood health issues that can have negative implications for adult health include the age at which **menarche** occurs in girls. Menarche indicates the beginning of a woman's reproductive life and coincides with the onset of menstruation. An association with menarche at age 12 or less with the risk of metabolic disease in early adulthood, breast cancer and reduced survival rate into old age has been identified. As menarche is occurring increasingly early, more girls will be exposed to these risks in the future (Rich-Edwards, 2002; Giles et al., 2010; United Nations Children's Fund, 2011b).

Ill health in childhood may also have socioeconomic consequences in adulthood; it can lead to lower educational attainment, an increased risk of unemployment in adult life, less likelihood of being a homeowner and reduced **social support** (Case et al., 2005; Kuh et al., 2005). However, recent studies have indicated that the role of childhood health problems in adult health and social pathways may have been overestimated. Nonetheless, even though these studies have led to arguments that the role of childhood illness is 'small', it is still acknowledged that it is 'non-trivial' (Palloni et al., 2009: 1579).

Undiagnosed Mental Health Problems

Although it is widely acknowledged that 'the majority of mental illnesses have childhood antecedents' (Royal College of Psychiatrists, 2010: 9), up to 70 per cent of children with diagnosable mental health disorders are undiagnosed and untreated. As a result, this group of children have an increased vulnerability to mental health problems later on in their lives (McCrone et al., 2008; Department of Health, 2011c). Aggressive behaviour in children (mentioned above) has been linked to problems in adolescence such as 'higher incidences of involvement with the youth justice system, gang and weapon carrying, smoking and anti-social behaviour' (Parentline Plus, 2010: 6). Abnormal levels of aggression in childhood that are not effectively treated are also associated with problems in adolescence and adulthood. Examples of these are the development of anti-social personality disorders, alcohol and drug misuse, criminality and unemployment (Parentline Plus, 2010).

Passive Smoking

In Chapter 2, we saw how smoking in pregnancy increases a baby's risk of mortality, bronchitis and pneumonia in the first year of life. Several other long-term effects to their health across the life course that have been identified, such as psychiatric problems in young adulthood and heart attacks and strokes in midlife, were also discussed. With reference to exposure to passive smoking during babyhood, this has been related to higher incidences of sudden death syndrome. In addition, it increases babies' and children's risk of dental caries, respiratory diseases, asthma, acute or chronic middle-ear diseases and slow lung growth. Furthermore, passive smoking in babies' and children has been linked to leukaemia, lymphoma, lung cancer and brain tumours. Clearly, the severity of some of these health problems means that they will inevitably impact on health and well-being at other life stages (Department of Health, 2009c; Brown et al., 2010b; Ortega et al., 2010; Tanaka et al., 2010).

How are you doing with your grid? Here are some suggestions about points that you could have included so far for you to check out.

Childhood influences	Outcomes in adolescence
Birth trauma	The effects of irreversible injuries to the skeleton, clavicle fracture, head trauma and perinatal asphyxia. Traumatic birth experiences can also lead to childbirth-related post-traumatic stress disorder in mothers. Amongst the outcomes of such disorders is an inability to bond with the child that has effects on psychological health and cognitive development
Maternal depression	Cognitive and emotional developmental problems as a result of the impact of maternal depression on a mother's parenting style

ACTIVITY 3.2

(Continued)

(Continued)

Childhood influences	Outcomes in adolescence
Undiagnosed mental health problems	Increased vulnerability to mental health problems. Untreated aggression in children has been linked to problems in adolescence such as involvement with the youth justice system, gang membership, weapon carrying, smoking, alcohol and drug misuse and anti-social behaviour
Passive smoking	Respiratory diseases and asthma in adolescence

Diet and Nutrition

Inadequate diets that contain an excess of fat and sugar intake and not enough fruit, vegetables and high fibre products can impair muscle and neurological growth and development in childhood. Poor nutrition in childhood can also lead to many physical and mental health problems in adulthood, such as high cholesterol, cardio-vascular diseases, diabetes, high blood pressure and depression (Desai, 2000).

Overweight and Obesity

Apart from the fact that obesity itself is a disease and is now the most common childhood disease in the developed world, overweight and obese children are at an increased risk of developing various health problems during their childhood years. These include orthopaedic conditions, bronchitis, Type 2 diabetes, low self-esteem, depression, behaviour problems and poor body image. Additionally, children who are overweight or obese are likely to experience decreased life satisfaction, poorer quality family relationships, higher school absenteeism and lower school performance. Over the course of their lives, obese children are at a greater risk of developing sleep apnoea, diabetes, hypertension, heart disease, liver disease and cancer (Brown et al., 2010c; Garthus-Niegel et al., 2010; Wijga et al., 2010); Padilla-Moledo et al., 2011). There is also increasing evidence that obesity in adulthood is associated with a loss of **health-related quality of life** in adulthood (Reilly, 2006; Minet Kinge and Morris, 2010).

Unfortunately, many children who are overweight or obese carry obesity into later life. As Figure 3.1 shows, when this occurs, it can cause chronic diseases in adulthood, for instance muscularskeletal disease, heart disease, some cancers, pulmonary disease, diabetes, strokes, high blood pressure, asthma, as well as mental illness such as mood disorders. The life-threatening consequences of these effects on health and well-being across the life course have led to fears that increasing obesity rates in childhood threaten 'to reverse the gains in longevity made during the last hundred years' and that 'today's children will die at a younger age than their parents will' (Finch and Searle, 2005: 122). Recent research has indicated that these risks may be higher for boys who are overweight or obese during childhood than for girls (Lawlor et al., 2010). Furthermore, some of the outcomes of being overweight or obese in childhood, such as higher school absenteeism and a lower school performance, have negative correlations with future educational and socioeconomic status that in turn increase the risks to health and well-being in adulthood (Finch and Searle, 2005; *Foresight Report*, 2007; Brown et al., 2010c; Sanderson et al., 2011).

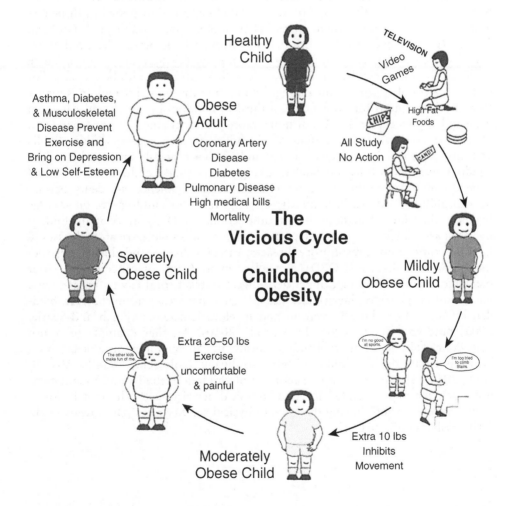

Figure 3.1   Childhood obesity and adulthood

Source: Statistics of Childhood Obesity, 2011: Health life tips from www.katrinatribute.info/statistics-of-childhood-obesity-is-getting-higher.html

Discussion Point

Look at Figure 3.1 again. How what is so-called 'The vicious cycle of childhood obesity' be broken?

Health Behaviour

Although children rarely have diseases associated with health behaviour, childhood is not only the first stage of accumulated exposure to poor health behaviours but is also 'a time when health behaviours become established' (Graham, 2009: 29), which shapes future health behaviours and outcomes. These points are demonstrated in Figure 3.1 in relation to obesity. Furthermore, there is much evidence that many children are learning less than optimal health behaviours. For instance, alcohol consumption amongst children in the United Kingdom is higher than in other countries; on average, a third of children in the United Kingdom drink at least once a week, with drinking more prevalent amongst boys than girls. Of further concern is the amount of alcohol consumed in one session. Public attention has turned to 'binge drinking' and this has certainly increased for older children over the past decade. Such drinking patterns make children in the United Kingdom more vulnerable to unsafe sexual behaviour, violence, accidents, permanent disabilities and death. Similarly, smoking rates for children are on average higher in the United Kingdom than in other countries. Daily smoking in children has been associated with psychological problems and smoking-related illnesses in later life, for example, respiratory diseases, vascular disease and chronic obstructive pulmonary disease (COPD), as well as many forms of cancers. The latter include cancers of the lung, upper aero-digestive tract (oral cavity, nasal cavity, nasal sinuses, pharynx, larynx and oesophagus), pancreas, stomach, liver, bladder, kidney, cervix, bowel, ovarian and myeloid leukaemia (Finch and Searle, 2005; Bradshaw et al., 2006; Peto et al., 2010). Another example of health behaviour is physical activity. Being physically fit can exert a favourable effect on health not only during childhood but also during adolescence (Padilla-Moledo et al., 2011). However, a large proportion of children in the United Kingdom do not reach the recommended levels of physical activity, with children in lower socioeconomic groups having the lowest physical activity rates (Drenowatz et al., 2010; Fisher et al., 2011).

Child Abuse

There is evidence that a substantial minority of children experience physical, emotional and sexual abuse (Larkin, 2009). Any form of child abuse significantly increases children's vulnerability to drug abuse, mental health problems, psychiat-ric disorders, offending and anti-social behaviour during childhood as well as into adulthood (Hooper, 2005; Jackson and Scott, 2006; Jonas, et al., 2011). A very recent study found an association between childhood abuse and sexual risk-taking behaviour in middle age (Wilson and Widom, 2011). Bullying by peers is often classified as a form of child abuse, too, and can lead to self-harm, social anxiety, depression and poorer educational attainment. Bullied children are also at risk of substance abuse in adolescence and young adulthood and of being victimised in later life. As it is estimated that up to 50 per cent of children are bullied at some point during their childhood, many children are at risk of these negative conse-quences. Moreover, those who are bullies in childhood are more likely to exhibit anti-social behavior in adulthood and have problems with maintaining stable rela-tionships and long-term employment (Hooper, 2005; Bradshaw et al., 2006; Kim, et al., 2011). Nonetheless, there are those who argue that the level of bullying is exaggerated and that learning to cope with a certain amount of unpleasant behav-iour from other children helps develop resilience and healthy social and emotional skills for adult life (Gill, 2007).

Finished your grid? Now compare the risks that are likely to affect health and well-being in adolescence that you have identified with those in Table 4.1 in Chapter 4. Are there any differences? If so, why do you think that these differences exist?

ACTIVITY 3.3

Is it all down to the Parents?

As we have already established, the extent to which risks to health and well-being do result in adverse outcomes depends on a range of, often interacting, influ-ences. These need to be considered in order to gain a deeper understanding of the extent to which childhood can shape an 'individual's health and well-being across their whole life' (Graham, 2009: 26). In the discussions above, we saw how par-ents influence their children's diet, weight, health behaviour and exposure to passive smoking. Indeed, parents exert a critical influence over health and well-being during childhood and there is a substantial body of evidence about the different ways in which parents contribute to childhood health and well-being. For instance, the way in which a child is parented has been found to have a sig-nificant effect on many aspects of their mental health in childhood and later life. Reference was made in the previous section as to how impaired mother–child attachment as a result of childbirth-related post-traumatic stress disorder and postnatal depression can cause cognitive and emotional developmental problems. The importance of children experiencing a secure, warm, intimate, rewarding and responsive relationship with their parents for the quality of their mental health during other life stages has been established across many academic disciplines for some time. These disciplines include child development, psychiatry, psychology and sociology (Bowlby, 1965; Parkes et al., 1991; Wadsworth and Compas, 2002; Barlow and Svanberg, 2010). Research continues to support this view; studies have shown that children who do not form secure parental attachments are more likely to develop substance abuse problems in adolescence and unsuccessful relationships in adulthood (Rutger and van den Eijnden., 2007; Green, 2010). A recent study by Landau et al. (2010) found that children who receive inadequate responsivity, particularly to negative emotions or distress, from their parents are at greater risk of developing attention deficit hyperactivity disorder (ADHD) than children who have more responsive interactions with their parents. Other current research has adopted an interdisciplinary approach and linked our earliest relationships and the behaviour within them to the development of our neurological system that in turn determines future emotional well-being (Gerhardt, 2006). A specific example can be found in Leach's work (2010), when she cites evidence that being left to cry causes babies acute and continuing distress that in turn causes their adrenal glands to flood the body and brain with the stress hormone, cortisol. High levels of cortisol that build up over time can affect a baby's brain development and alter brain stress thresholds with the result that a child may become liable to anxiety and depression.

The nature of the parental relationship and parental mental health are also important influences on a child's mental health. Conflict between parents can increase the risk of a child developing an anti-social personality disorder, and witnessing domestic violence in the home triples the likelihood of children having conduct disorders. Research has also shown that young adults who experience aggressive conflict in their own relationships often attribute this to violence in their parental backgrounds (Green, 2010). Children of parents who separate are four times as likely to develop emotional disorders as those in families who stay together. However, paternal involvement with their children after separation can help protect against later mental health problems (Meltzer et al., 2009; Parentline Plus, 2010). With reference to parental mental health, poor parental mental health is associated with a four to five times increased risk of mental illness in childhood, adolescence and adulthood (Parentline Plus, 2010; Garber et al., 2011). Furthermore, losing a parent during childhood and teens to suicide is a catalyst for a range of major psychiatric disorders and suicide (Kuramoto et al., 2010).

Further evidence about how parents influence children's health and well-being comes from research that shows how they shape their health behaviour. The extent to which childhood health behaviour has implications for children's long-term health and well-being has already been established. One of the most notable examples is parental smoking; children are more likely to smoke if their parents smoke (Department of Health, 2009c; Brown et al., 2010b). Studies have found that parents are also the most important influence on children's attitudes to alcohol. Although parents do not specifically teach their children about the health consequences of drinking, their own drinking behaviour conveys messages about alcohol consumption (Eadie et al., 2010; Valentine et al., 2010; Sondhi and Turner, 2011). Another very recent study has shown that 'tough love' parenting, combining consistent warmth and discipline, is the most effective parenting style to prevent unhealthy relationships with alcohol from childhood right into the mid-thirties age range (Bartlett et al., 2011). In addition, whilst the alarming increases in obesity have been attributed to multiple factors, several studies have highlighted the extent to which parents play a key role in determining whether their child is overweight or obese. This is because they influence both the quality and quantity of their children's dietary intake and their levels of physical activity. With reference to physical activity specifically, higher levels of physical activity have been found amongst children whose parents encourage their participation in outdoor and sporting activities, are physically active themselves, do not have high levels of TV viewing and whose mothers do not work full-time. Furthermore, higher parental TV viewing has been associated with an increased risk of high levels of TV viewing for both boys and girls (Brown et al., 2010c; Hart et al., 2010; Jago et al., 2010; King et al., 2010; Hendrie et al., 2011; Miller, 2011). The extent to which parents recognise that their child is overweight is yet another factor in child obesity. Many parents of overweight children fail to acknowledge that they have a weight problem and therefore do not ensure that they make appropriate adjustments to their diet and physical activity levels (Lynch et al., 2010; Sealy, 2010). In some cases, this can be attributed to the different cultural values about what is an attractive and healthy body shape; some groups, such as Black Africans, favour fuller body shapes and identify heavy child body shapes as healthy (Harrison et al., 2011b).

As you can see from the above discussions, it can be argued that many of the ways in which parents influence their children's health and well-being during childhood and in the longer term are not always within their immediate control, for example if they are mentally unwell themselves. Other important factors over which parents may have limited control also operate at an individual level. These include the manifestations of a child's personality and the number of friendships in childhood. The role of the former in adult health was addressed in Chapter 1. The latter have been linked to health disparities in adulthood; those who have a higher number of such friendships report better self-rated health in middle age (Kubzansky et al., 2009; Almquist, 2011). However, as indicated in our exploration of the risks to health and well-being during infancy and childhood, the extent of parental influence is shaped by the wider social environment. Although features of this environment mentioned were socioeconomic factors, ethnicity, gender and poverty, much of the research has focused on poverty and deprivation. Whilst parents often try to protect their children from some of the impacts of childhood poverty, children living in poverty still suffer more health problems than those who do not live in poverty (Bradshaw et al., 2006; Palloni et al., 2009). More detailed evidence of the role of poverty comes from studies of specific aspects of childhood health. Not only do the poorest children have the highest mortality rates, but they also have the highest rates for acute and chronic illness, respiratory problems, mental ill health, behavioural problems, obesity and both accidental and **non-accidental injury**. Childhood poverty also has negative effects on cognitive and social development (Graham and Power, 2004; Beresford et al., 2005; Graham, 2009; Parentline Plus, 2010; Marmot Review Team, 2011). In addition, poverty in childhood has been linked to increased risks of cardiovascular disease, obesity and Type 2 diabetes in adulthood, as well as to lower educational attainment, employment and socioeconomic status (Case et al., 2005; Kuh and Ben-Shlomo, 2005; Graham, 2009).

Explanations of the long-term effects of poverty on children vary. Life course research has shown how exposure to social and economic adversity in childhood negatively affects multiple biological systems. If this exposure continues into adulthood, these effects accumulate with the result that biological functioning in middle and later adulthood is compromised. Those who experience improvements in their social and economic circumstances from childhood to adulthood were found to have similar physiological and biological functioning in midlife and older age to those who had been persistently socially and economically advantaged during their life course. This suggests that upward mobility in childhood and early adulthood has potential protective effects for physiological function in middle and late adulthood (Gruenewald et al., 2012). As explained in Chapter 1, those working within the life course perspective who adopt an epidemiological approach to health and well-being emphasise that it is the timing of exposure to events that determines their eventual impact on our health (Kuh and Ben-Shlomo, 2005; Lynch and Davey Smith, 2005). They use the concepts of 'critical periods' or 'sensitive periods' to denote those points in our lives when exposure to particular events or risks have more lasting or lifelong effects. This epidemiological approach has been applied to poverty in childhood. Studies have shown that the effects of poverty may be magnified at particular times in childhood, for example during periods of important childhood social transitions, such as starting school (Lynch and Davey Smith, 2005).

The poorest children's living conditions and the fact that they experience more of the risks that can compromise health and well-being (as outlined in the previous section) have been the focus of other explanations about the effects of poverty on children (Davey Smith and Ebrahim, 2002; Marmot Review Team, 2011). With reference to living conditions, cold housing and fuel poverty are usually a consequence of growing up in poverty. Cold housing has been found to have significant negative effects on 'infants' weight gain, hospital admission rates, developmental status, and the severity and frequency of asthmatic symptoms' (Marmot Review Team, 2011: 9). In relation to the risks discussed that can compromise health and well-being, children in the poorest families are more likely to have a mother who suffers from postnatal depression, have either never been breastfed or only breastfed for a short time, have an unhealthy diet, be obese, be exposed to passive smoking and to experience abuse (Jackson and Scott, 2006; Alwan et al., 2010; Brown et al., 2010a; Department of Health, 2011c). Poverty has also been shown to 'penetrate deep into the heart of childhood' and permeate through 'to the most personal often hidden aspects of disadvantage associated with shame, sadness and the fear of social difference and marginalisation' (Ridge, 2011: 73). Some groups of children are far more vulnerable to poverty than others. These are homeless children, some ethnic minority groups and those in particular types of families such as asylum seeker and lone parent families, large families and families in which people have a disability. Therefore the health and well-being of these children is at greater risk than other children living in less severe poverty (Beresford et al., 2005; Brewer et al., 2006).

Other features of the wider social environment that have been identified are the relationship between food advertising on obesity in children, preschool education, and access to healthy food outlets (supermarkets and greengrocers) and unhealthy outlets (takeaways and convenience stores) around homes and schools (Keller and Schulz, 2010; D'Onise et al., 2011; Harrison et al., 2011a). The impact of changes in our social environment on children's health and well-being cannot be ignored either; cuts in public spending have recently resulted in children undertaking less physical activity at school (Helm, 2010). A very recent report has shown that whilst the materialist culture in the United Kingdom has led to a parental compulsion continually to buy new consumer goods for their children, children often feel that family time is more important (United Nations Children's Fund, 2011a). Rising unemployment rates means that one in six children now live in a workless household. Parental unemployment is associated with a two to three times increased risk of the child developing emotional and/or conduct disorders. In addition, higher unemployment means that more children will experience poverty and its associated impact on their health and well-being. As the full effects of the economic downturn and reductions in public sector spending in the United Kingdom have yet to be experienced, there will be worse to come (Meltzer et al., 2003; United Nations Children's Fund, 2010). Consequently, there may be decreases in child health and well-being and, as demonstrated, this will also have implications for the health and well-being throughout the life course of those currently in this age cohort.

Improving Health and Well-Being in Childhood

As we saw in Chapter 1, the value of a life course perspective on health and well-being is increasingly being advocated at policy level. Although this has led to a recognition of the relevance of prevention interventions at each life stage, there has been an emphasis on using preventative strategies in childhood in order to improve health and well-being. This is because this life stage is now seen as being pivotal to health and well-being throughout the life course, and hence, early interventions are essential. The extracts in Box 3.1 from various documents produced within the last couple of years demonstrate how this view is now a common theme in the approaches being advocated for improving the health and well-being of the population.

Box 3.1 The best start in life

Giving every child the best start in life is crucial to reducing health inequalities across the life course. The foundations for virtually every aspect of human development – physical, intellectual and emotional – are laid in early childhood. What happens during these early years (starting in the womb) has lifelong effects on many aspects of health and well-being – from obesity, heart disease and mental health, to educational achievement and economic status. To have an impact on health inequalities we need to address the social gradient in children's access to positive early experiences. Later interventions, although important, are considerably less effective where good early foundations are lacking. (Marmot, 2010: 16)

'[S]ince the majority of lifetime mental illnesses develop before adulthood', prevention targeted at children and adolescents 'can generate greater personal, social and eco-nomic benefits than interventions at any other time in the life course'. (Royal College of Psychiatrists, 2010: 25)

There is 'overwhelming evidence that children's life chances are most heavily predicated on their development in the first five years of life. It is family back-ground, parental education, good parenting and the opportunities for learning and development in those crucial years that together matter more to children than money, in determining whether their potential is realised in adult life. The things that matter most are a healthy pregnancy; good maternal mental health; secure bonding with the child; love and responsiveness of parents along with clear boundaries, as well as opportunities for a child's cognitive, language and social and emotional development. Good services matter too: health services, Children's Centres and high quality childcare. Later interventions to help poorly performing children can be effective but, in general, the most effective and cost-effective way to help and support young families is in the earliest years of a child's life. (Field, 2010: 5)

'Taking better care of our children's health and development could improve edu-cational attainment and reduce the risks of mental illness, unhealthy lifestyles, road deaths and hospital admissions due to tooth decay. (Department of Health, 2010b: 5)

You can see from the above that health and well-being is set in the context of the overall quality of life chances and that improving health and well-being in childhood involves improving many aspects of children's lives. This is also reflected at policy level in the development of integrated policies based on the premise of maximising health over the entire life cycle (Blackwell et al., 2001; Case et al., 2005). However, the scale and nature of interventions that have been introduced have varied considerably; whilst some are implemented at international and national levels, others are community, school and/or family based. Parenting interventions in particular have proliferated because of the many benefits that have been attributed to them (Barlow and Svanberg, 2010). Whilst these benefits are summarised in the following extract, cost–benefit analyses of sustained parenting interventions in the United States also provide strong evidence of their economic benefits (Reynolds et al., 2011):

> Parenting interventions promote better parental mental health, better outcomes for the child, including school behaviour and attainment and reduce the risk of a lifetime course of poor health and outcomes, including criminality and anti-social behaviours. It reduces the take-up of risky behaviours including smoking, alcohol and substance misuse. It also has the power to break negative intergenerational cycles by improving parenting style and skills for the current as well as next generation. (Parentline Plus, 2010: 8).

Other policies have attempted to address social inequalities in childhood, most notably those caused by poverty. Although 'the last ten years have seen an unprecedented commitment to tackling child poverty in the United Kingdom, with the aim of eliminating it in 2020' (Graham, 2009: 30), the targets set are unlikely to be met and the strategies used have been criticised for their lack of sustainability. Moreover, an increase in child poverty over the next decade is predicted (Brewer et al., 2012). A case has been made for developing an alternative strategy to abolish child poverty that advocates preventing poor children from becoming poor adults by adopting a life course approach. This is based on the evidence about the importance of the preschool years to children's life chances. It is argued that government policy and spending within this alternative strategy should focus on developing children's capabilities in the early years as this is the period when it is most effective to do so. The emphasis should be on the provision of high-quality integrated services aimed at supporting parents and improving the abilities of our poorest children. Those advocating such a strategy maintain that these measures will greatly enhance the poorest children's 'prospects of going on to gain better qualifications and sustainable employment' and 'change the distribution of income by changing the position which children from poor backgrounds will be able to gain on merit in the income hierarchy' (Field, 2010: 6).

There have also been interventions targeted at specific aspects of health and well-being in childhood. These are often highly innovative and examples include interventions to reduce passive smoking, smoking, obesity and to improve mental health (*Foresight Report*, 2007; Ortega et al., 2010; Royal College of Psychiatrists, 2010; Department of Health, 2011c).

Read through the following extract from a newspaper article and then think about the questions below:

CIGARETTES 'TO BE SOLD IN PLAIN BROWN PACKS': TOBACCO COMPANIES MAY BE FORCED TO USE UNGLAMOROUS PACKAGING IN BID TO STOP CHILDREN BEING ATTRACTED TO SMOKING

The government is considering forcing tobacco companies to package their cigarettes in plain brown wrappers in a bid to de-glamorise smoking and stop young people taking up the habit. The Health Secretary, Andrew Lansley, is investigating the viability of introducing what would be one of the most radical public health measures ever implemented in the United Kingdom. Senior doctors welcomed the potential ban on colours and logos on packets and said it could prove as effective as the 2007 public smoking ban. However, Ministers are likely to face a legal challenge if they go ahead. 'We have to try new approaches and take decisions to benefit the population. That's why I want to look at the idea of plain packaging,' said Lansley. 'The evidence is clear that packaging helps to recruit smokers, so it makes sense to consider having less attractive packaging. It's wrong that children are being attracted to smoke by glitzy designs on packets.' Lansley stressed that the need to prevent children from starting to smoke in the first place was his main motivation for taking seriously a policy which the tobacco industry fears would be hugely damaging. 'We would prefer it if people did not smoke, and adults will still be able to buy cigarettes (even if plain packs come in), but children should be protected from the start' he said. (Campbell, 2010)

1   Do you think that the proposal to package cigarettes in plain brown wrappers will make smoking less attractive to children?
2   What other action needs to be taken in order to reduce smoking rates among children?
3   What strategies would you include in a life course approach to children's smoking?

Conclusions

One of the main purposes of this chapter was to explore the claim that childhood is 'an unparalleled time during which external influences, both good and bad, can influence an individual's health and well-being across their whole life' (Graham, 2009: 26). This has involved an examination of the evidence about the risks to health and well-being that can occur in childhood and the extent to which they threaten health and well-being during childhood and in other stages in the life course. The discussions about the implications of these risks, together with recognition of the importance of this life stage for health and well-being throughout the life course at national and international policy level, show that it is not unreasonable to conclude that there is a considerable body of evidence to support Graham's view of childhood. The next chapter will address health and well-being in adolescence as adolescence inevitably follows childhood and is also one of the other life stages that Graham identifies as being an 'unparalleled time' in relation to health and well-being across the life course. However, the life course perspective argues that health outcomes are cumulative from conception, through to infancy, childhood, adolescence, adulthood and old age. Therefore, Graham's claim cannot fully be assessed without consideration of the ongoing impact of the aforementioned risks in the other life stages. Consequently, we will continue to reflect on the significance of pregnancy, childhood and adolescence in subsequent chapters in the book.

Summary

- Whilst the overall health of children in the United Kingdom dramatically improved throughout the last century, the prevalence of mental health disorders has increased and new health issues amongst children have also been identified. Examples of these are the rises in chronic illnesses and obesity rates
- Prenatal influences can only provide a partial understanding of childhood health and well-being. A more complete understanding can be gained from an exploration of the risks to health and well-being that can occur in childhood. These are birth itself, breastfeeding, maternal depression, childhood illnesses, undiagnosed mental health problems, passive smoking, diet and nutrition, obesity, health behaviour and child abuse
- These risks can compromise health and well-being during childhood and some of them can be a threat to health and well-being in other stages in the life course
- Although parents exert a critical influence over health and well-being during childhood, there are some important factors over which they may have limited control. These include certain features of the wider social environment
- Initiatives have aimed to reduce the risks that occur during childhood that threaten health and well-being in this life stage and at other life stages
- The adoption of a life course approach to health and well-being at policy level has led to the emphasis on using preventative strategies in childhood in order to improve the health and well-being of the general population. Whilst some policies have been introduced at international and national levels, others are community, school and/or family based

Further Study

There are several very useful publications based on surveys of children's health and well-being. An example is J. Bradshaw and E. Mayhew (eds), *The Well-Being of Children in the UK*, 2nd edn (London: Save the Children Fund, 2005). If you need information to make international comparisons in childhood health and well-being, it is worth looking at:

(Continued)

(Continued)

- Bradshaw, J., Hoelscher, P. and Richardson, D. (2006) *Comparing Child Well-Being in OECD Countries: Concepts and Methods*. Florence: United Nations Childern's Fund (UNICEF).
- United Nations Children's Fund (UNICEF) (2007) *Child Poverty in Perspective: An Overview of Child Well-Being in Rich Countries, Innocenti Report Card* 7. Florence: United Nations Children's Fund Innocenti Research Centre.
- United Nations Children's Fund (UNICEF) (2010) 'The children left behind: a league table of inequality in child well-being in the worlds rich countries'. (Florence: United Nations Children's Fund Innocenti Research Centre.
- For a more in-depth exploration of socioeconomic factors, see H. Graham (ed.), *Understanding Health Inequalities*, 2nd edn (Maidenhead: McGraw Hill, 2009). Journal articles written by Hilary Graham will also be very helpful.

4

Health and Well-Being in Adolescence

Overview

- Introduction
- Health and well-being in adolescence
- Pre-adolescent life
- Risks to health and well-being during adolescence
- Risk mediators in adolescents' health and well-being
- Mediating the mediators in adolescent health and well-being
- Conclusions
- Summary
- Further study

Introduction

Although there are debates about the existence of adolescence as a universal phenomenon and when it commences and ends, it is widely recognised that adolescence is a phase that is separate from childhood. There are also clear changes in health and well-being in adolescence (Green, 2010; Platt, 2011). For instance, we saw in Chapter 1 that rates of acute and chronic illnesses start to increase after the age of 16. When the data about health and well-being in adolescence is disaggregated, it also shows that there can be a gulf in experience between younger and older adolescents. Such findings have led to distinctions between 'early adolescence' and 'late adolescence' being made (United Nations Children's Fund, 2011b). Whilst it is recognised that the concept of adolescence is problematic and that such distinctions are somewhat arbitrary, in this chapter 'adolescence' will be regarded as the second decade of life. Reference to experiences that are common in the early and later stages of this period will be made as necessary.

This chapter will continue the examination of the view introduced at the end of Chapter 2 that like *in utero* development and childhood, adolescence is another 'unparalleled' life stage 'during which external influences, both good and bad, can influence an individual's health and well-being across their whole life' (Graham, 2009: 26). It will start by providing an overview of adolescent health and well-being and then move on to an exploration of health and well-being at this life stage from a life course perspective. The first part of this exploration will address the extent to which adolescent health and well-being is shaped by pre-pregnancy, prenatal and childhood experiences and simultaneously show how health outcomes are cumulative from conception. The discussions will then move on to the possible risks to health and well-being during adolescence as well the many ways in which these in themselves and in some cases in combination with factors in earlier life, can affect health and well-being in adulthood and old age. The next section will look at the sorts of variables that can modify the impact of these risks. This is followed by a reflection on policies that have been developed to improve adolescent health and well-being. When the material presented inevitably overlaps with that in other chapters, this will be acknowledged.

Health and Well-Being in Adolescence

Adolescence is typically conceptualised in the Western world as a time of disruption and turmoil, with terms such as 'storm and stress' being used in the literature to convey its nature. The fact that it involves rapid and dramatic physical and psychological changes that are part of the transition from childhood to adulthood cannot be ignored. Whilst physical changes usually start between the ages of ten and fourteen, girls tend to experience these on average 12 to 18 months before boys. This period is often referred to as 'early adolescence', and begins with a growth spurt followed by the development of the sex organs and secondary sexual characteristics. Although the internal changes are less obvious, they are equally profound; research has shown that 'the brain undergoes a spectacular burst of electrical and physiological development. The number of brain cells can almost double in the course of a year, while neural networks are radically reorganised' (United Nations Children's Fund, 2011b: 6). 'Late adolescence' is said to occur between 15 and 19 years of age. By this time, most of the major changes have occurred but the body does continue to develop. For instance, the brain is still reorganising itself, with the result that capacity for analytical and reflective thought is greatly enhanced (Green, 2010; United Nations Children's Fund, 2011b).

Adolescents may appear healthier than other age groups and to some extent this is supported by the statistics available on adolescent health and well-being, both nationally and internationally. Examples include the way in which their asthma and acute illness rates are lower than during childhood, they experience fewer chronic illnesses and use services less frequently than adults. They may also give the impression of being less worried about their health. Moreover, there is some evidence of a rise in levels of health and well-being amongst adolescents. Nonetheless, the external changes that occur during adolescence can be a source of anxiety and the range of changes described above inevitably has implications for health and well-being at this life stage. Indeed, over 50 per cent of adolescents visit their general practitioner at least once a year, and around 30 per cent have some type of, albeit minor, health problems. In addition, it is a time when certain acute and chronic conditions start. These include acne, scoliosis (curvature of the spine) and Type 1 diabetes. The latter peaks between the ages of 12 and 14 (Beresford et al., 2005; Coleman et al., 2007; Helms, 2007; Blanchflower and Oswald, 2008; United Nations Children's Fund, 2011b).

With reference specifically to mental health problems, these are more common in adolescence than in childhood and up to a quarter of adolescents experience 'distress or dysfunction' (Pilgrim, 2007: 194). Although the numbers affected have been rising since the Second World War, suicide rates in young people have declined significantly over the decade (Pilgrim, 2007; Biddle et al., 2008). Overall, girls have fewer psychological and mental health problems during adolescence. Although some problems, such as emotional and behavioural problems are generally becoming much more prevalent, there are marked gender differences in the types of mental health problems experienced by adolescents; girls are more prone to anxiety, depression and eating disorders such as **anorexia nervosa** and **bulimia nervosa**, whereas boys are more likely to have conduct disorders. Whilst boy's suicide rates are also four times higher, three times more girls than boys are involved with self-harming behaviour (Coleman, 2007a; Royal College of Psychiatrists, 2010; Darlington et al., 2011; United Nations Children's Fund, 2011b).

There are several adolescent health and well-being issues that are currently of particular concern. The frequency of young people cutting themselves appears to be increasing. Prevalence estimates vary between one in twelve and one in fifteen (Hall and Place, 2010). Another serious threat to health and well-being in adolescence is the continued rise in the numbers of adolescents who are obese; 25 per cent of adolescents are now classified as overweight or obese and this figure is predicted to increase. The fact that the numbers of those who are diagnosed with eating disorders are increasing – and many cases still remain undiagnosed – has caused similar levels of concern. A further issue is adolescent sexual health; there has been a dramatic increase in **sexually transmitted diseases (STDs)** (also known as sexually transmitted infections) (STIs)), particularly amongst young men. Although other European countries have experienced rises in some types of sexually transmitted infections (such as chlamydia), the overall number of sexually transmitted infections is higher in the United Kingdom (Coleman, 2007b:

86; Faulkner, 2007; Lowry et al., 2007). In connection with adolescent sexuality, there is ongoing concern about the **teenage birth rate**. Despite the fact that teenage conception rates have declined since 1998 and about only half of these lead to a maternity, rates of teenage births are still the highest in Western Europe and the United Kingdom is second only to the United States in the developed world (Coleman, 2007b; Office for National Statistics, 2009b).

Discussion Point

To what extent do you think that adolescence in the Western world is a time of 'storm and stress'?

Pre-Adolescent Life

In the next two sections, we will continue our exploration of health and well-being across the whole lifespan from a life course perspective with specific reference to adolescence. Given the way in which this perspective emphasises the cumulative nature of health outcomes from conception through to old age, this section will focus on the role of pregnancy, prenatal and childhood influences on health and well-being at this life stage. Those discussed in Chapters 2 and 3 are summarised in Table 4.1. Once again, as health and well-being across the life course is such a dynamic area of research, this summary cannot be completely comprehensive. It has been compiled with the intention of demonstrating the potential cumulative effects in adolescence of risks to health and well-being that occur in pre-adolescent life.

Table 4.1 clearly demonstrates the way in which risks to health and well-being can accumulate prior to adolescence. However, it does not reflect the way in which the outcomes of the risks in childhood for health and well-being in adolescence are shaped by a range of interacting influences. Those discussed included parenting style and features of the wider social environment, such as socioeconomic factors, ethnicity, gender and poverty. Similarly, there are factors that can offset some of the negative outcomes that also need to be considered in an exploration of adolescence from a life course perspective. Examples given were regular physical activity, a child's personality and improved social and economic circumstances. As well as acknowledging these interacting influences and variables that can have 'protective effects' (Bryant et al., 2003: 363), in order to progress our examination of the importance of this life stage for health and well-being across the whole life course we need to discuss the sorts of factors identified in the literature that are most likely to compromise health and well-being during adolescence and their implications for later life. These are addressed in the next section.

Table 4.1 The impact of pre-adolescent risks to health and well-being in adolescence

Pre-pregnancy influences	Outcomes for health and well-being in adolescence
Maternal pre-pregnancy weight below 50 kg	This can lead to low birth weight, which in turn can result in a range of adverse health outcomes in adulthood, such as cardiovascular diseases, hypertension and diabetes

Fetal exposures	
Low-quality maternal diet	Poor fetal growth and low birth weight that can result in cardiovascular diseases, hypertension, obesity and diabetes
Obesity in pregnancy	Increases risk of abnormality
Risks associated with certain foods such as uncooked meat, fish, eggs	Hydrocephalus (water on the brain), brain damage, epilepsy, deafness, blindness and growth problems
Maternal alcohol consumption	Physical and neurodevelopmental problems as a result of fetal abnormalities. Examples of these problems are facial deformities, physical and emotional developmental problems, memory and attention deficits, as well as cognitive and behavioural problems
Prenatal stress	As this can lead to low birth weight, the risks of cardiovascular diseases, hypertension and diabetes in adolescence are higher. Some studies have also found links with increased vulnerabilities to learning impairments and psychopathology
Smoking and regular exposure to smoke-filled environments in pregnancy	Increased risk of respiratory diseases and asthma
Uncontrolled Type 1 or Type 2 diabetes	The effects of congenital malformation

Childhood risks	
Birth trauma	The effects of irreversible injuries to the skeleton, clavicle fracture, head trauma and perinatal asphyxia. Traumatic birth experiences can also lead to childbirth-related post-traumatic stress disorder in mothers. Amongst the outcomes of such disorders is an inability to bond with the child, which has effects on psychological health and cognitive development
Maternal depression	Cognitive and emotional developmental problems as a result of the impact of maternal depression on a mother's parenting style
Undiagnosed mental health problems	Increased vulnerability to mental health problems. Untreated aggression in children has been linked to problems in adolescence, such as involvement with the youth justice system, gang membership, weapon carrying, smoking, alcohol and drug misuse and anti-social behaviour

(Continued)

Table 4.1 *(Continued)*

Childhood risks	Outcomes for health and well-being in adolescence
Passive smoking	Respiratory diseases and asthma in adolescence
Smoking	Psychological problems, respiratory diseases, vascular disease and chronic obstructive pulmonary disease (COPD), as well as many forms of cancer. The latter include lung, upper aero-digestive tract (oral cavity, nasal cavity, nasal sinuses, pharynx, larynx and oesophagus), pancreas, stomach, liver, bladder, kidney, cervix, bowel and ovarian cancer, as well as myeloid leukaemia
Diet and nutrition	An inadequate diet in childhood that contains an excess of fat and sugar intake and not enough fruit, vegetables and high-fibre products can impair muscle and neurological growth and development in adolescence
Overweight and obesity	Increased risk of developing orthopaedic conditions, bronchitis, Type 2 diabetes, low self-esteem, depression, behaviour problems and poor body image. As a result of being overweight or obese in childhood, adolescents are also likely to experience decreased life satisfaction, poorer quality family relationships, higher school absenteeism and lower school performance
Child abuse	Increased vulnerability to drug abuse, mental health problems, psychiatric disorders, offending and anti-social behaviour
Being bullied	Bullied children are at risk of substance abuse in adolescence
Insecure parental attachments and ineffective parenting	Poorer mental health and emotional well-being, as well as developing a substance abuse problem and an unhealthy relationship with alcohol in adolescence
Poor parental mental health	This is associated with a four to five times increased risk of mental illness in adolescence

Risks to Health and Well-Being During Adolescence

The first two of these risks are the experience during adolescence of chronic illnesses and mental illness, respectively. We will then move on to the implications of risk-taking behaviours for adolescent health and well-being. As you will be aware, adolescence is a time of experimentation, 'testing the boundaries' and risk-taking. Much of the research carried out nationally and internationally has focused on the extent to which this risk-taking approach features strongly in many health and lifestyle behaviours that develop during adolescence. Taken to extremes, these behaviours can be fatal, as evidenced by the statistics that show that young males between 16 and 24 account for almost 60 per cent of driver fatalities even though they only represent 10 per cent of licensed drivers. More generally, behaviours that are deemed to be a risk to health in adolescence have been defined as 'voluntary behaviours that threaten the well-being of teenagers' (Leishman and Moir, 2007: 1), and typically include inadequate physical activity, obesity, poor nutrition, sexual risk-taking and substance abuse. Although such risk-taking declines during late adolescence and rarely results in lifestyle-related diseases during this stage, the accumulated exposure to the threats that it poses to health and well-being can have adverse consequences later on in life. These consequences may also be severe and lifelong. As some risk-taking behaviours developed during adolescence are also continued into later life, their impact on adult morbidity and mortality is further exacerbated (Helms, 2007; Leishman and Moir, 2007; Fisher and Gerein, 2008; Musacchio amd Forcier, 2008; United Nations Children's Fund, 2011b). Therefore, in order to reflect their widely recognised significance for health and well-being, these adolescent behaviour patterns will be the focus of the rest of the discussions about the sorts of factors that can affect health and well-being during and after adolescence. Although the risk-taking behaviours identified in the literature do tend to occur together and may have different impacts on different individuals (Coleman et al., 2007; Wills, 2008), each type is discussed individually below, together with their general consequences.

The grid set out below uses the same format as that in Table 4.1. As you read through the rest of this section, try to identify any risks that are likely to affect health and well-being in young adulthood. Make a note of them on the grid. This activity is designed to help you continue to develop your ability to interpret the findings about health and well-being at a particular life stage from a life course perspective.

ACTIVITY 4.1

Risks in adolescence	Outcomes for health and well-being in young adulthood

Chronic Illness in Adolescence

As mentioned above, there have been rapid increases in the incidence of chronic illnesses between early and late adolescence for both boys and girls. In addition to their physical and psychological effects, those who experience any chronic illness at this life stage are denied experiences and opportunities that serve a developmental function in adolescence. For example, they may miss out on experiencing sexual relationships. They may also become isolated from their social networks because friendships become harder to develop and sustain. This can result in social isolation in adulthood. In addition, adolescents with a chronic illness can find themselves unable to pursue educational and employment opportunities that can reduce their future employment prospects (Helms, 2007; Grinyer, 2007, 2009; Eilertsen et al., 2011).

We will use the examples of diabetes and cancer to illustrate the more specific health problems of chronic illnesses in adolescence (Coleman et al., 2007; United Nations Children's Fund, 2011b). Taking the example of diabetes first, the health problems that this chronic illness brings are:

> an increased risk of a range of potentially devastating complications including blindness, renal failure, cardiovascular disease and diabetic neuropathy. Psychological problems, such as depression and anxiety, are also much more common in people with diabetes compared to those without. (Lloyd and Skinner, 2009: 128)

When diabetes is well managed and complications are prevented, these long-term effects are considerably reduced (Lloyd and Skinner, 2009). However, the risks of death from diabetes are higher in adolescence and early young adulthood than in other life stages, particularly for females. A recent study found that females between the ages of 15 and 34 with Type 1 diabetes were 9 times more likely to die than other women of the same age. Males in the same age group were 4 times more likely to die if they had the condition. For Type 2 diabetes, the figures are 6 and 3.6 times, respectively (NHS Information Centre for Health and Social Care, 2011).

With reference to the example of cancer, although this is relatively uncommon amongst adolescents, studies show that when compared to children, incidence rates have increased over the past decade. They also rise during the teenage years and into young adulthood. In addition to the effects of cancer on their physical health, a cancer diagnosis impacts negatively on many aspects of adolescents' health and well-being. Cancer and its treatment inevitably bring disempowerment, a loss of independence, changes in physical appearance (for example, hair loss, weight gain and scars from surgery) and an underlying anxiety about long-term health. Adolescence is a time when issues such as independence, appearance and planning for the future are very important. Hence, adolescents with cancer are particularly sensitive to these consequences of their illness, and studies show that they often experience considerably reduced levels of self-confidence and emotional well-being that can last for several years following diagnosis and treatment.

Sadly, in addition to having to endure the aforementioned health and well-being problems, many adolescents with cancer do not recover; survival rates for cancer in adolescence are very poor and it is 'the most common cause of death' in this age group 'exceeded in incidence only by accidental death' (Grinyer, 2007: 1). This has been attributed to a range of factors that include the fact that during this life stage there tends to be less parental involvement in health matters, adolescents typically lack awareness of symptoms and are unwilling to seek medical advice. Misdiagnosis is also common because symptoms are frequently unspecific and can be lifestyle related, such as 'tiredness'. Those who do survive into adulthood often experience ongoing anxiety and fertility issues that in the longer term affect well-being and life planning. Furthermore, some adolescent cancers and/or their treatments 'can lead to secondary cancer or treatment-related cancer in later life' (Grinyer, 2009: 6) (Grinyer, 2007, 2009; Crawshaw and Sloper, 2010; Tromp et al., 2011).

Mental Illnesses

As half of all mental illnesses begin by the age of 14 and three-quarters by the mid 20s, together with young adulthood, adolescence is a time in the life course when mental health problems are most likely to develop. However, adolescent mental health problems are often undiagnosed and untreated. This has been attributed to a variety of reasons; studies have shown that adolescent turmoil is rarely recognised by others. Many adolescents who experience distress are also unlikely to seek help because they are reluctant to articulate their feelings to professionals. In addition, they consistently report poor communication between themselves and health professionals when discussing mental health concerns (Harvey et al., 2007; McCrone et al., 2008; Parentline Plus, 2010).

Poor mental health in adolescence not only impacts on this life stage but also has lifelong implications for health and well-being. Its adverse effects are compounded by the aforementioned under-diagnosis and low treatment rates. Those who suffer from mental health problems during adolescence are more likely to miss school and have physical health problems, fewer friends -and more limited social networks. The experience of mental ill health during adolescence has also been linked to various difficulties in adulthood. These include major depression, suicidal behaviour, alcoholism, anti-social personality disorders, drug misuse, as well as decreased employment opportunities, relationship problems, lower income, lower owner-occupation rates and increased probability of criminal activity (Beresford et al., 2005; Bradshaw et al., 2006; Coleman, 2007a; Pilgrim, 2007; Kerr and Capaldi, 2011). Indeed, there is some evidence to suggest that mental disorders in adolescence have more adverse effects on longer-term quality of life than physical illnesses experienced at this life stage (Chen et al., 2006).

The major eating disorders – anorexia nervosa and bulimia nervosa – have serious health consequences during adolescence and in adulthood. Although there are arguments that, for some adolescent sufferers, anorexia nervosa represents stability and control, they do suffer from anaemia, frequent infections, extreme fatigue and hormonal abnormalities. The latter in turn can lead to retarded growth and irregular or absent menstruation. Bulimia is associated with rupture of the oesophagus, mineral deficiency and dehydration, hormonal imbalances, major depression and suicide. In about 10 per cent of cases, anorexia sadly leads to multiple organ failure and death. Indeed, despite the fact that bulimia nervosa is not generally as dangerous to health, both conditions are responsible for a higher number of deaths than any other psychiatric disorder. Whilst the prevalence of eating disorders decreases towards the end of adolescence and many adolescents do make a full recovery, sufferers are at risk of heart and gastrointestinal diseases, infertility, nerve damage and osteoporosis in adulthood (Fox et al., 2005; Faulkner, 2007; McCrone et al., 2008; Treasure and Friederich, 2009; Abebe et al., 2012).

Inadequate Physical Activity

There has been a general decline in engagement in physical activity, particularly amongst girls, and many adolescents now lead relatively sedentary lives (Lowry et al., 2007). Appropriate levels of physical activity during adolescence have been found to be beneficial in many different ways. As well as improving physiological fitness, the more immediate benefits include reductions in levels of anxiety, stress and depression, and enhanced mood and self-esteem. Regular physical exercise also has a longer-term antidepressant effect and can delay the onset of certain chronic diseases in adulthood such as coronary heart disease, various cancers, hypertension, diabetes and osteoporosis. In addition, physical activity has been found to increase the likelihood of adolescents engaging in health promoting behaviours. However, these benefits are not universally applicable; overtraining at a young age can cause muscle development problems in skeletal frameworks that are not fully mature. There are also psychological disorders associated with exercise. One of these is **Female Athlete Triad (FAT)**. This is most common amongst young women who take part in sports that emphasise low body weight (for example, ballet dancing and ice-skating) and is the physical manifestation of a pathological pursuit of exercise regimes. It is often coupled with an inappropriate diet. However, establishing a physically active lifestyle during adolescence has been shown to increase the likelihood of adherence to healthy exercise routines throughout the life course (Nabkasorn et al., 2005; Lowry et al., 2007; Tassitano, et al., 2010; Delisle et al., 2010).

Poor Nutrition

High levels of vegetable and fruit consumption in adolescence are linked to lower risks of cancer and coronary heart disease in later life. Surveys of the number of vegetable and fruit portions consumed daily by adolescents in the United Kingdom show that whilst girls have a better record than boys, the overall figures for adolescents are lower in comparison with other countries. Further questions about the quality of their diet have been raised by evidence that adolescents in the United Kingdom rank amongst the worst countries for consumption of energy-dense food, such as sweets and soft drinks. Nonetheless, concerns about the quality of adolescent nutrition are not unique to the United Kingdom; a recent study showing that adolescents in the United States get a fifth of their calories from fast food and that only a minority of fast food outlets meet good nutrition criteria received much attention (Finch and Searle, 2005; Roehr, 2010).

Overweight and Obesity

A further consequence of reduced physical rates is that adolescents today expend between 600 and 700 less calories than their counterparts 50 years ago. This reduction in average energy expenditure has contributed to the increase in obesity rates amongst adolescents referred to above (Reilly, 2006; Faulkner 2007). Studies show that the physical and psychological health and well-being of overweight and obese adolescents is threatened both during and after their adolescence. During adolescence, they are at an increased risk of developing orthopaedic conditions, bronchitis and Type 2 diabetes. They are also likely to suffer from low self-esteem and depression as well as experience poorer quality family relationships, bullying at school and lower school performance. Such outcomes can have detrimental effects on important developmental processes, too. When adolescent obesity continues into adulthood, it can increase the risks of sleep apnoea, high blood pressure (a major cause of strokes), high cholesterol levels, hearing loss and mental illness. In addition, obesity in adolescence has been linked to many chronic diseases in adulthood that can potentially shorten the lifespan. These include heart disease, liver disease, cancers and diabetes (Finch and Searle, 2005; Faulkner, 2007; *Foresight Report*, 2007; Brixval, et al., 2011; Ecob et al., 2011; Fonseca et al., 2011; Patton et al., 2011). Not surprisingly, there is evidence that obesity is also associated with loss of health-related quality of life in adulthood (Minet Kinge and Morris, 2010).

How are you doing with your grid? Here are some suggestions about points that you could have included so far, for you to check out.

ACTIVITY 4.2

Risks in adolescence	Outcomes in young adulthood
Chronic illnesses	Emotional and developmental problems, serious medical conditions, ongoing anxiety, reduced employment prospects, secondary cancer or treatment-related cancer in later life, fertility issues that in turn affect well-being and life planning, higher risks of mortality than in other life stages

(Continued)

(Continued)

Risks in adolescence	Outcomes in young adulthood
Poor mental health	Major depression, suicidal behaviour, alcoholism, anti-social personality disorders, drug misuse, decreased employment opportunities, relationship problems, lower income, lower owner-occupation rates and increased probability of criminal activity
Anorexia nervosa and bulimia nervosa	Heart and gastrointestinal diseases, infertility, nerve damage and osteoporosis
Poor nutrition	Increased risk of cancer and coronary heart disease in later life
Overweight and obesity	Risk of developing sleep apnoea, high blood pressure (a major cause of strokes), high cholesterol levels, mental illness, heart disease, liver disease, cancer and diabetes as adults. In addition, there is evidence that obesity in adulthood leads to a loss in health-related quality of life

Sexual Activity

The life course approach argues that adolescent sexuality must be seen as a developmental process. Active exploration of sexual well-being during adolescence is simply part of the more general exploration of identity, values, goals and behaviour that takes place at this life stage, all of which contribute to health and well-being at later stages in the life course. However, adolescent sexuality becomes more of a cause for concern when it stops being 'exploratory sexuality that ultimately contributes to positive sexual identity and competence', and 'significantly increases risk of harm' (Halpern, 2010: 6). Collecting data about adolescents' sexual activity is problematic because of ethical issues and the fact that it is often dependent on retrospective accounts of sexual activity. Nonetheless, studies have identified some of the ways in which it can be a risk to health and well-being. For instance, adolescents in this country become sexually active at an early age; whilst there is now a possible stabilisation of age of first intercourse, it is lower in the United Kingdom than in other European countries. In addition, they tend to have more sexual partners and to change those partners more frequently than older age groups. Although use of at least one form of contraception has increased, the use of condoms having increased the most, inconsistent use of contraception and an increase in the number of sexual partners have resulted in the higher rates of sexually transmitted diseases reported at the beginning of the chapter. Genital chlamydia is the most common sexually transmitted infection amongst adolescents

but an increasing number are being reported as having infectious syphilis, gonor-
rhoea, genital herpes, genital warts and the **Human Immunodeficiency Virus
(HIV)** (Beresford et al., 2005; Coleman, 2007b; Halpern, 2010). Sexually transmitted infections can cause pelvic inflammatory disease and recurrent episodes of
infection. The asymptomatic nature of some of these infections and the fact that
teenagers are reluctant to seek help about their sexual health means that they are
liable to remain undetected, putting the health of those infected at greater risk.
As sexually transmitted infections are also associated with stigmatisation, prom-
iscuity and embarrassment, they can impact on emotional well-being. In addition,
there are longer-term consequences for those who contract sexually transmitted
diseases in adolescence; they are at risk of ectopic pregnancy, miscarriage, infertility and chronic illnesses (including some cancers) in later life. With reference to
HIV specifically, although treatable, it is still incurable and causes **Acquired
Immune Deficiency Syndrome (AIDS)**. This is a condition that results in the progressive failure of the immune system that in turn leads to life-threatening infections
and cancers. Furthermore, any babies born to HIV sufferers may be premature,
have low birth weight, experience neonatal complications or be stillborn. Such
threats to health and well-being both during and following adolescence may
increase because of the strain that the rising incidence of sexually transmitted
infections has placed on services and the resultant delays in the availability of
appointments and treatment (Coleman, 2007b; Harvey et al., 2007; Leishman,
2007; Health Protection Agency, 2009).

Unplanned pregnancies are another highly significant consequence of adolescents'
early, unprotected sexual activity. As mentioned earlier in the chapter, the under-20
birth rate in the United Kingdom is the second highest in the developed world.
Whilst there is some data about teenage fathers, this is limited to their support needs
and most of the studies that have been carried out have focused on teenage mothers.
These show that teenage pregnancies are associated with poor outcomes for both the
mother and her child; teenage mothers are vulnerable to certain medical problems
during pregnancy and childbirth, such as anaemia, hypertension, prolonged, difficult
or premature delivery and postnatal depression. Their babies are more likely to be
low birth weight, have higher infant and child mortality rates and not be breastfed.
Postpartum, they often experience a range of problems that affect both their own
and their children's lives. Examples are physical and mental health problems, poor
educational, social and economic opportunities, parenting problems, domestic
violence and drug dependency. Children of teenage mothers are also more likely to
experience childhood disadvantage and twice as likely to become teenage parents
themselves. However, research has found that these consequences vary with the age
that pregnancy occurs and that for some teenage mothers their child gives them
much satisfaction and a sense of direction in life. Hence, the impacts of teenage
motherhood on health and well-being are not totally negative (Beresford et al.,
2005; Coleman, 2007b: 90; Leishman, 2007).

There are further risks to health and well-being when an unplanned teenage
pregnancy ends in abortion. Half of all teenage conceptions end in abortion and
the figures are higher for pregnancies in early adolescence than in later adolescence.
Although there are more risks of complications, such as excessive bleeding, when

an abortion is carried out in unsafe and illegal conditions, teenagers generally have lower rates of morbidity and mortality from induced abortion than older women. Nonetheless, teenage abortion can lead to depression in both the mother and the father. It can also impact on the mother's health and well-being in the longer term in that it has been shown to lead to an increased chance of breast cancer, pelvic inflammatory disease, depression and the contraction of viral hepatitis (Spencer, 2001; Leishman, 2007).

Substance Abuse

Whilst definitions vary, substance abuse is most often associated with a maladaptive but non-dependent use of nicotine, recreational drugs and alcohol. Whilst early research indicated that use of such substances during adolescence reflected psychological maladjustment, it is now acknowledged that some experimentation is functionally necessary and helps adolescents to gain resources to develop a healthy lifestyle. Indeed, 'statistically speaking', substance abuse is 'fairly normal among adolescents' (Rutger et al., 2007: 108). Furthermore, studies have shown that experimental substance use has several benefits in terms of identity formation, short-term relief from stress and negative feelings, increased sociability and the facilitation of romantic experiences. Moreover, there is evidence that experimental substance use does not persist into adulthood. Frequent excessive use is linked to starting such experimentation in early adolescence and poor psychological adjustment. It also has numerous harmful effects that range from a deterioration in youngsters' relationships with their parent to increased risks of depression and **suicidal ideation**, as well as permanent impairment of the explosive brain development that takes place in adolescence, referred to above. Another consequence of such problematic use is its trajectory; it is usually nonlinear, rising rapidly through adolescence and only flattening out through young adulthood. Evidence about the harmful effects of substance use in adolescence has led some to argue that they outweigh the benefits that have been identified (Hallfors et al., 2004; Rutger et al., 2007; Guo et al., 2010; Eschmann et al., 2011; United Nations Children's Fund, 2011b). In the rest of this section we will examine the patterns of non-dependent smoking, use of recreational drugs and drinking in adolescence and the possible risks to health and well-being.

Smoking

It is estimated that about 20 per cent of adolescents smoke regularly but there is evidence that their actual smoking rates may be higher than reported (Fuller and Sanchez, 2010). The numbers increase with age, with boys being more likely to smoke than girls. When international comparisons are made, smoking rates amongst adolescents in the United Kingdom are higher than in many other countries. Despite the fact that some studies show that smoking provides adolescents with a means to gaining control of feelings and situations, it has been associated with psychological problems and smoking-related illnesses in later life (Finch and Searle, 2005; Bradshaw et al., 2006; Nilsson and Emmelin, 2010). These include not only lung cancer but also other types of cancers such as cancer of the upper aero-digestive tract (oral cavity, nasal cavity, nasal sinuses, pharynx, larynx and oesophagus), pancreas, stomach, liver, bladder, kidney, cervix, bowel, ovary and myeloid leukaemia. With reference to lung cancer specifically, there is evidence that smoking initiation in adolescence increases the risk of lung cancer independently of the amount smoked or duration of smoking. Other smoking diseases that are recognised as being related to smoking are respiratory diseases, vascular disease and chronic obstructive pulmonary disease (COPD) (Wiencke, 1999; Peto et al., 2010).

Recreational Drug Use

Although rates of recreational drug use increase between 11 and 16 years of age, it is relatively uncommon before the age of 16 compared to the period from 18 to 25. There has also been a slight reduction in illegal substance misuse in recent years (Jotangia et al., 2010). Negative effects associated with specific drugs have been identified, such as the way in which cannabis use contributes to school dropout. However, recreational drug use does have positive effects in that it can enhance social competence. More problematic is a progression from recreational to regular drug use as this is not only likely to lead to serious and/or persistent offending but also to a drug use career (Bradshaw et al., 2006; Legleye et al., 2009; Järvinen and Ravn, 2011).

Alcohol Abuse

The number of adolescents who report drinking alcohol at least once a week is increasing and up to one third binge drink, with 6 per cent reaching the threshold of having an alcohol-related **substance use disorder**, including alcoholism (Rutger et al., 2007). Drinking alcohol is more prevalent in boys than in girls. Adolescent alcohol consumption is a problem across Europe, but as with adolescent smoking rates, international comparisons show that the United Kingdom does not compare favourably; a higher proportion of adolescents in the United Kingdom than those in other countries drink at least once a week (Finch and Searle, 2005; Donath et al., 2011; Regis, 2011).

There is evidence that adolescents drink because of the perceived positive consequences. Hence they drink 'because they want to have fun, to have a good time with friends and/or a partner or to feel good and not to become involved in fights or car accidents' (Rutger et al., 2007: 119). Nonetheless, adolescent alcohol consumption in general is associated with many negative consequences that include lower academic performance and several known risks, such as traffic and other accidents, aggression, sexual assaults and unsafe sexual behaviour. The risks are even greater when it comes to binge drinking. It is now well established that binge drinking at any stage of the life course has many adverse outcomes. These include fractured friendships, accidents, law-breaking (especially assault, violence and vandalism), arguments, neglect of obligations, suicide, as well as increased risks of unplanned sex, unprotected sex, unplanned pregnancies and HIV infection. Physiologically, binge drinking causes changes in blood glucose levels, white blood cell activity, blood pressure, female reproductive hormone levels and cardiac rhythm. In the longer term, it has also been linked to psychological problems, irreversible brain damage, cognitive impairments and **ischaemic heart disease**. Studies of adolescents specifically have shown that regular binge drinking has serious implications for health and well-being during adolescence and in adulthood. During adolescence it can cause unsafe sexual behaviour, irreversible brain damage, cognitive impairments, traffic accidents and other types of accidents and violent behaviour as well as lead to suicide and the consumption of other psychotropic substances. With reference to health and well-being in adulthood, regular binge drinking profoundly increases the risks of liver disease, infertility and developing an alcohol-related disorder and/or alcoholism (Finch and Searle, 2005; Coleman, 2007b; Connor et al., 2010; Balsa et al., 2011; United Nations Children's Fund, 2011b).

ACTIVITY 4.3

Finished your grid? Now compare the risks that are likely to affect health and well-being in adolescence that you have identified with those in Table 5.1 in Chapter 5. Are there any differences? If so, why do you think that these differences exist?

Risk Mediators in Adolescents' Health and Well-Being

The above discussions highlighted the way in which the impact of the risks to health and well-being in adolescence is unpredictable and mediated by variables, one of the most important being gender. Studies of adolescent health and well-being have identified a range of potential variables and emphasise the importance of seeing them not only as interacting with each other but also as being 'embedded in a whole system of other events and behaviours, all of which influence each other' throughout adolescence (Coleman et al., 2007: 8). Moreover, this body of research has demonstrated the ways in which some of these variables can have 'protective effects' (Bryant et al., 2003: 363) and offset exposure to certain risk factors. It has also been argued that adolescents differ in their reactions to risks depending on their own biographies. Examples of these are personality profile (for example, self-efficacy and impulsivity), genetic characteristics and resources that adolescents develop as a result of life experiences (including taking risks). These sorts of factors interact, too, and have different effects at different times. Hence, 'pursuits or activities which are healthy for one person can be unhealthy for another and without any health consequences for a third' (Coleman et al., 2007: 8) (Bryant et al., 2003; Kuh and Ben-Shlomo, 2005; Coleman, 2007b; Coleman et al., 2007). Therefore, as part of our assessment of the significance of the experience of adolescence for future health and well-being, we need to examine these variables in more detail. As gender has already been mentioned, we will start with this variable and then move on to other key influences that have been identified in the literature.

Gender

Read through the following newspaper article. As you read, think about the following questions:

1   What does it tell us about the ways that gender influences the health and well-being of teenage girls?
2   What other sorts of influences does it discuss?

The issues raised by these questions are addressed in the rest of this section of the chapter.

Twice as many girls are suffering 'teenage angst' as boys, according to research [by the thinktank Demos] that suggests growing up in Britain is toughest on young women ... and there is evidence that they have become more miserable over the past three years. The problem is said to be particularly acute for those from lower socioeconomic backgrounds ... . The research follows recent studies which suggest that girls also lead unhealthier lifestyles than boys, skipping meals to lose weight, as well as drinking and smoking too much. Girls are more anxious than boys about their appearance, careers and a celebrity culture that places a premium on good looks. Some young women also feel burdened by an increased expectation to continue to move into areas of work that had been male-only. Teenagers also suffer peer pressure to have sex earlier than ever before. ... Meanwhile, the Director of Public Prosecutions has warned that girls aged 16 to 19 are now the group most at risk from domestic violence.

Julia Margo, deputy director of Demos, said the thinktank's report, *Through the Looking Glass*, provided evidence that 'Growing up has always been tough, but our research shows that this generation of teenagers has more reason to wallow and fret than previous generations. It is definitely tougher to grow up in Britain as a girl, and it is harder having to do it now than it has been in recent years.'

Analysis of Department for Education statistics by Demos reveals the extent to which self-esteem differs between teenage girls and boys. There are around 5.5 million teenagers in the United Kingdom and just over half are girls. A significantly higher proportion

(Continued)

(Continued)

> of girls aged 14 to 15 report feeling 'worthless', 'unhappy or depressed' or 'low in confidence', compared with boys. The proportion of teenage girls who report feeling worthless 'rather more than usual' and 'much more than usual' was twice the number of teenage boys. Most strikingly, almost a third of girls report feeling unhappy and depressed 'rather more than usual' and 'much more than usual', which was also twice as much as boys. More than a fifth of teenage girls report they have been losing confidence 'rather more than usual' and 'much more than usual', compared with just over one in 10 teenage boys. (Boffey, 2011)

There are conflicting views of the exact relationship between gender and health and well-being in adolescence. On the one hand, there are those who point to the evidence to suggest risk-taking behaviour is less common amongst girls and that in general they are significantly more successful in making the transition to adulthood. Their outcomes, especially in education and youth offending, reflect this. They also do better in their exams and more of them go to university (Pesa et al., 2001; Coleman, 2007a). However, the above article indicates that there may be a different relationship between gender and health and well-being in adolescence; according to the recent study about teenage boys and girls to which it refers, girls are increasingly more likely to be unhappy, have a poorer diet, smoke and drink. Several of these findings are supported by other studies. These show that around one in three girls aged between 15 and 16 admits that she binge drinks and that there is now a new breed of adolescent drinkers – young women who drink very heavily and have a tendency towards violence. Furthermore, British teenage girls do not compare well with their European counterparts in that they have worse rates of binge drinking, worse levels of physical inactivity and more frequent incidences of teen pregnancy (Desai, 2010; Darlington et al., 2011).

Studies show that there are many other factors that play an important role in the relationship between gender and health and well-being in adolescence. For instance, girls who experience an early menarche are more likely to affiliate with older adolescents and engage in risky behaviour, such as smoking and drinking (Bradshaw et al., 2006; Gaudineau et al., 2010). The article above also makes several references to ways in which contemporary culture impinges on teenage girls' health and well-being and as this is also one of the other key influences on adolescent health and well-being in general, we will now explore this in more depth.

Culture

The report on which the article is based concludes that 'this generation of teenagers faces a more difficult environment in which to make the transition into adulthood' (Darlington et al., 2011: 9). Several features of this 'more difficult environment' have been identified as being particularly significant in the studies that have been carried out. These include social, economic and technological developments. For instance, the fact that adolescents today expend between 600 and 700 fewer calories than their counterparts 50 years ago was mentioned in the previous section. This has been attributed in part to mass car-ownership, computer, Internet and television use. Consequently, for many adolescents, 'physical exercise is no longer considered a necessity but may represent a lifestyle choice' (Lowry et al., 2007: 20). Increased drinking amongst adolescents has been linked to the drinking culture in the United Kingdom (Desai, 2010). Moreover, the latter is seen as a cause of changes in the drinking culture in Mediterranean countries, such as France, which have led to sharp rises in 'le binge-drinking' (Allen, 2011: 25) amongst the youth. The greater emphasis on assessment and exams in schools, the changing job market and increasing difficulties in finding stable employment because of the global economic recession have been blamed for the psychological and mental health problems amongst adolescents (Bradshaw et al., 2006; Coleman, 2007a; McCrone et al., 2008; Royal College of Psychiatrists, 2010). Some of the mental health problems more commonly experienced by girls have been found to be fuelled by cultural constructions of femininities (Landstedt et al., 2009).

The role of the media cannot be ignored when discussing cultural influences on adolescent health and well-being. Indeed, the media has been found to contribute to adolescents' high levels of sexual experience and sexual risk-taking (Ward and Friedman, 2006; Coleman, 2007b). There are also arguments that the media obsession with weight and body shape and use of stereotypes of feminine beauty plays a significant role in the incidence of eating disorders, such as anorexia and bulimia (Faulkner, 2007; Bendelow, 2009; United Nations Children's Fund, 2011b).

Whilst the power of youth subcultures to shape adolescent behaviour has been recognised since the 1950s, over the past couple of decades this body of research has been extended to include the role of peer and friendship group pressure in adolescent sexual risk-taking, smoking and drinking behaviours. Both national and international studies show that peer groups are extremely influential. Interestingly, although they usually circumvent parental control and result in an increase in such behaviours, some peer groups can have very positive effects. For example, adolescents who belong to a sports team have 'reduced lower levels of alcohol consumption' (Percy et al., 2011: 6) (Finch and Searle, 2005; Kwansa, 2007; Green, 2010; Pollard et al., 2010; McVicar, 2011; Percy et al., 2011).

As we all know, culture is not homogeneous and most Western societies now comprise many different cultural, ethnic and religious groups. These in turn have been found to influence health and well-being in adolescence. For example, young people from Black backgrounds have lower levels of mental disorder than other ethnic groups (10 per cent compared to 16 per cent), with those from an Indian background having the most significantly lower levels (3.5 per cent). Evidence from studies that have looked at adolescent health behaviours across ethnic and cultural groups shows that Black teenagers in general compare the most favourably. This indicates that cultural backgrounds can have 'protective effects'. Religiosity has also been found to have protective qualities in relation to mental distress, substance use and sexual activity (Nonnemaker, et al., 2003; Coleman, 2007a; Boardman and Alexander, 2011; Donath et al., 2011).

Parental Influences

Although the influence of parents on their children in adolescence is not as strong as in childhood, the style of parenting and family life in adolescence impacts on health and well-being in many ways (Mayhew et al., 2005). Adolescents whose parents are authoritative but also accepting of their need for psychological autonomy and are warm, supportive, accepting and uncritical, are more likely to have higher levels of self-esteem, as well as lower levels of depression, anxiety and behaviour and substance abuse problems (Steinberg, 2001; Quilgars et al., 2005; Walton and Flouri, 2010; Bartlett et al., 2011). In contrast, those who experience harsh, punitive parenting are more likely to develop depression and a range of emotional, behavioural (including delinquency) and substance abuse problems (Wadsworth and Compas, 2002; Bartlett et al., 2011; Roche et al., 2011). With reference to family life, family arguments and family conflict have been linked to aggression, anxiety and depression (Wadsworth and Compas, 2002). Other aspects of family life that have been found to influence health and well-being are parental separation and/or divorce, the death of a parent and/or being cared for in a looked-after setting. The last two of these are associated with higher rates of mental health disorders (Gibbs et al., 2005; Economic and Social Research Council, 2011).

The issue of parental influence in adolescence has been fiercely debated; there are arguments that much of what has been attributed to parental influence is actually genetic, and when adolescents are influenced by the environment it is peers who are more likely to have the strongest influence, not parents. However, such views have been criticised because they ignore the substantial literature about the extensive role that parents do play in the socialisation of their children. Furthermore, parents directly and indirectly manage their children's choices about friendships during childhood that in turn predispose them to certain peer relationships during adolescence. Therefore, even if peers do exert a significant influence in adolescence, they arguably often reflect parental values and inclinations (Harris, 1998; Steinberg, 2001).

Further persuasive evidence about the extent of parental influence during adolescence comes from the body of literature about how they shape health behaviour at this life stage. For example, parental physical activity levels have been linked to adolescents' activity levels (Martín-Matillas et al., 2010). In relation to substance use, parents own substance habits and their parenting practices, such as their supervision and support of their children, have been found to be highly influential (Kwansa, 2007; Rutger et al., 2007; Sondhi and Turner, 2011). Whilst there are several theories about the causes of eating disorders and it is now accepted that there are multiple interacting causes, some researchers still maintain that particular features of certain families 'predispose young people to the development of anorexia' (Faulkner, 2007: 71); these features include lack of conflict resolution, marital disillusionment, covert coalitions, over-protectiveness and rigidity. Nonetheless, it has been argued that these features are not unique to families with an anorexic member but are characteristic of the family of anyone who has some form of psychiatric probem (Faulkner, 2007). Similarly, different types of families, such as **reconstituted families** and **lone parent families** have been found to be associated with higher rates of risk-taking behaviours (Finch and Searle, 2005; Coleman et al., 2007).

Poverty and Social Disadvantage

The impact of poverty on health and well-being in adolescence is unequivocal. Some of the most notable examples are the ways in which poverty increases the risk of chronic illnesses, psychological problems, mental health disorders, suicide, teenage motherhood and more problematic substance use that is likely to lead to serious and/or persistent offending (Wadsworth and Compas, 2002; Beresford et al., 2005; Bradshaw et al., 2006; Coleman et al., 2007). Some of the specific consequences of poverty, such as cold housing and fuel poverty, have also been linked to poorer adolescent health and well-being (Marmot Review Team, 2011). The close relationship between poverty and low socioeconomic position means that the effects of belonging to a lower socioeconomic group are often similar. For instance, higher levels of unhappiness, mental disorders and teenage pregnancies, as well as overweight and obesity rates, have been found amongst young people in lower socioeconomic groups (Quilgars, 2005; Kwansa, 2007; Darlington et al., 2011). Moreover, there are inverse social gradients for fresh fruit and vegetable consumption and physical activity levels (Finch and Searle, 2005; Coleman, et al., 2007; Morgen et al., 2010). Whilst previous literature has shown that adolescents in lower socioeconomic groups are more likely to engage in substance abuse, there is now growing evidence that adolescents in high socioeconomic groups are also at high risk of substance abuse (Humensky, 2010). Some of these outcomes, such as lower levels of physical activity, are more pronounced in boys than in girls (Pabayo et al., 2011).

Other features of adolescents' circumstances mediate some of these problems; an adolescent from a low socioeconomic group who is in looked-after settings, in custody or in prison faces a considerably elevated risk of having a mental health disorder (Neale, 2005; Coleman, 2007a). In contrast, ethnicity mitigates the impact of poverty on teenage motherhood (Beresford et al., 2005; Coleman et al., 2007). More generally, parenting and the quality of family relations can reduce some of the worse effects of poverty and social disadvantage in adolescence (Bradshaw et al., 2006). Furthermore, studies that adopt a life course approach to health and well-being show that the effects of poverty and social disadvantage are cumulative and can lead to higher illness rates (such as cardiovascular disease, obesity and Type 2 diabetes), offending, drug and alcohol abuse in adulthood, as well as reduced employment and earnings prospects (Bradshaw et al., 2006). Hence, the role of prenatal and childhood poverty and social disadvantage need to be taken into consideration in any assessment of the impact of these influences on health and well-being in adolescence (Graham, 2007; Platt, 2011).

Discussion Point

What evidence is there in the above discussions of the different influences of:

- interacting with each other?
- being 'embedded in a whole system of other events and behaviours, all of which influence each other' (Coleman et al., 2007: 8)?
- having 'protective effects' (Bryant et al., 2003: 363)?

Mediating the Mediators in Adolescent Health and Well-Being

As we have seen, the evidence linking early circumstances and adult health and well-being is very complex. Many studies have been carried out in order to find appropriate interventions to reduce the continuities in disadvantage during adolescence. These have used a variety of methodologies and addressed many different issues. The latter include mental health, eating disorders, education, sex education, smoking and drinking, youth offending and youth unemployment. A wide range of often highly innovative community, school and home based strategies have been trialled and advocated. Examples are interventions for developing self-esteem, promoting resilience and improving access to reproductive healthcare services (Harvey et al., 2007; Fisher and Gerein, 2008; Gretchen and Dulmus, 2010; Hogan et al., 2010; Wheeler, 2010).

There is now national and international recognition of the importance of investing resources in the second decade of life aimed at improving health and well-being across the life course. This recognition includes the need to prioritise the development and dissemination of effective policies so as to address adolescent health and well-being in order to maximise the personal, social and economic benefits of these policies over a lifetime (Darlington et al., 2011; United Nations Children's Fund, 2011). Therefore, we need to continue to carry out systematic research that takes into account young peoples' views and is thoroughly evaluated so that there is a robust evidence base for future interventions (Royal College of Psychiatrists, 2010; Sainsbury Centre for Mental Health: Rethink, 2010). A review of the relevant literature also strongly indicates that in order to address the myriad of interacting influences on adolescent health and well-being, interventions need to involve a number of sectors and focus on individual, political, economic, social and cultural factors. In addition, serious consideration needs to be given to the provision of more training in adolescent health and well-being for health professionals (Macfarlane and McPherson, 2007; Kidger et al., 2009; Hughes et al., 2011).

Conclusions

As well as examining some of the key issues in adolescent health and well-being, this chapter has discussed a range of factors that can potentially have negative effects on health and well-being during adolescence and in subsequent life stages. It has also explored the literature in relation to the variables that can shape the nature of the outcomes of these factors in the shorter and the longer terms. Whilst there is evidence of the role of some internal influences (such as personality and genetic characteristics), it is clear that 'external influences, both good and bad' in adolescence 'can influence an individual's health and well-being across their whole life' (Graham, 2009: 26). Therefore, this evidence, in combination with that presented in Chapters 2 and 3 on prenatal health and childhood, indicates that it would appear that Graham's view is well-supported by the research that has been carried out to date. The extent to which Graham's description of these life stages as having 'unparalleled' significance in relation to an individual's health and well-being across their whole life will be further discussed in the chapters on young adulthood, middle age and older age. It is to young adulthood that we now turn.

Summary

- Although adolescents may appear statistically healthier than other age groups, they are increasingly suffering from mental health problems, their obesity rates are rising and there has been a dramatic increase in sexually transmitted infections (STI) in this age group
- Prenatal and childhood factors have a significant influence on adolescents' health and well-being. Identified threats during adolescence include cancer, mental illness and risk-taking behaviours involving inadequate physical activity, obesity, poor nutrition, sexual risk-taking and substance abuse
- The accumulated exposure to these threats can have adverse consequences for health and well-being in later life that may also be severe and lifelong
- There are several known mediators in the risk to adolescents' health and well-being. These are gender, culture, parental influence and poverty and social disadvantage
- These mediators all interact with a variety of other factors and in some cases can protect adolescents from exposure to certain risk factors
- The value of investing in adolescence in order to improve health and well-being across the life course is now recognised nationally and internationally. Although a wide range of policies has been developed to date, there is an ongoing need for the development of effective and targeted policies

Further Study

Coleman, J., Hendry, L. and Kloep, M. (eds), *Adolescence and Health* (Chichester: John Wiley and Sons Ltd, 2007), contains several chapters that address a range of adolescent health and well-being issues and is also highly readable. The Joseph Rowntree Foundation has carried out some interesting studies on adolescent health behaviours. It is worth visiting their website (www.jrf.org.uk) for details of these.

If you have a particular interest in adolescent sexual activity and its implications for health and well-being, see: J.L. Leishman and J. Moir (eds), *Pre-teen and Teenage Pregnancy: A Twenty-First-Century Reality* (Keswick: M & K Publishing Ltd, 2007). National and international public health journals are also a useful source of information about adolescent health and well-being issues in general. For international comparisons of adolescent health and well-being, see United Nations Children's Fund , *The State of the World's Children 2011* (New York: United Nations Children's Fund, 2011b).

5

Health and Well-Being in Young Adulthood

Overview

- Introduction
- Health and well-being in young adulthood
- Life before adulthood
- Risks to health and well-being during young adulthood
- Influences on the risks to health and well-being during young adulthood
- Reducing the risks to health and well-being during young adulthood
- Conclusions
- Summary
- Further study
- Activity comments

Introduction

'Young adulthood' lacks the conceptual recognition of other life stages discussed in this book. For example, the terms 'first adulthood' or 'early adulthood' are often used interchangeably when reference is made to this period in our lives. However, it is normally regarded as spanning the third and fourth decades of our lives. The data about health and well-being across the life course presented in Chapter 1 showed that physical health starts to decline from late adolescence onwards. Although the incidence of mental health problems reduces throughout young adulthood until midlife, rates of mental distress are as high as those in old age.

Nonetheless, it is one of our healthiest and most energetic life stages and, overall, the stage of adulthood where we experience our best health and well-being. Ascertaining more detailed information about health and well-being in young adulthood per se is complicated by the fact that only a small proportion of the research carried out to date distinguishes between young and middle adulthood. This chapter will reflect the findings within the current body of knowledge about the health and well-being of those in their twenties and thirties as accurately as possible.

As in the other chapters in this book, we will assess the information presented in relation to the view introduced at the end of Chapter 2 that 'not only pregnancy but also childhood and adolescence' are 'an unparalleled time during which external influences, both good and bad, can influence an individual's health and well-being across their whole life' (Graham, 2009: 26). We will start by outlining some of the main issues about health and well-being during young adulthood. This life stage will then be explored from a life course perspective. The first part of this exploration will look at the effects of prenatal, childhood and adolescent influences on health and well-being in young adulthood. In view of the cumulative nature of these influences from previous life stages, this section of the chapter will be longer than the equivalent sections in the preceding chapters. The second part of the examination of health and well-being at this life stage from a life course perspective will focus on the possible risks to health and well-being during young adulthood and the extent to which these, alone and in combination with risk factors in preceding life stages, can impact on health and well-being in middle and old age. The influences on these risks to health and well-being in young adulthood will be addressed in the penultimate section. The chapter will end with an overview of the policies that have been aimed at improving health and well-being in young adulthood. Any overlaps with material presented in other chapters will be acknowledged as appropriate.

Health and Well-Being in Young Adulthood

The literature indicates that the first few years of young adulthood represent an extended period of development as the transition from adolescence and adulthood is completed and crucially important choices regarding relationships, work and lifestyle are made. Complex and dramatic neurobiological and psychosocial changes also occur during this transition. These subside as young adults enter their thirties. Around this time, too, life becomes more serious and is often characterised by 'settling down', which involves being less mobile and an increased investment in work, family, friends, community activities and values. Nonetheless, such refocusing of priorities brings new stresses that emanate from high levels of financial and emotional commitments. Other differences between early and later young adulthood that have been identified relate to biological function, cognition, strength and physical performance; these peak from 20 to 35 years of age and then wane thereafter (Green, 2010; Rugg, 2010).

Evidence about these phases has led to the use of the term 'sub-phases' of young adulthood and they have been the subject of much theorising. For instance, Levinson (1978) put forward a model based on the 'seasons of early adulthood'. These comprised the early adult transition, the age 30 transition, the settling down phase followed by the midlife transition. However, Levinson's model has been criticised because of its rigidity and the fact that the sample he used in his research was all-male. Subsequently, there has been more of an emphasis on the fluidity of the 'sub-phases' in young adulthood, as well as the way in which they vary not only between individuals, depending on the route that they take through adulthood, but also according to a number of social, cultural and historical indices. Factors contributing to their fluidity in the twenty-first century include the current prolonged transitioning into adulthood (because of changes in waged work and age of leaving home, for example), the expansion of education and increasing longevity, that have arguably rendered the age norms for major life events highly elastic (Beckett, 2009; Green, 2010; Platt, 2011).

Whatever the debates about these 'sub-phases', health and well-being across young adulthood does change. For instance, mental health disorders, particularly schizophrenia and eating disorders, as well as suicide rates, are higher amongst those in their early twenties than later on at this life stage (Lowry et al., 2007; Eckersley, 2009; Rogers and Pilgrim, 2010). Life satisfaction had been found to decrease throughout young adulthood until the mid to late forties, when it reaches a minimum (Blanchflower and Oswald, 2008). However, it has recently been argued that this is only correct under untestable conditions (de Ree and Alessie, 2011). Some general patterns in health and well-being have also emerged from the research into young adulthood. One example is mortality rates; in developed countries, mortality rates for young adults are typically very low and people at this life stage are less affected by naturally occurring disease and disabilities than are older age groups (Green, 2010). With the exception of testicular cancer, cervical cancer, and Hodgkin's lymphoma, cancer is much less common in this group of adults. Nonetheless, there has been a rise in the number of cancers diagnosed in young adulthood over the past decade (Grinyer, 2007).

There are several health issues amongst young adults that are becoming causes for concern. These are their rising diabetes and obesity rates and the fact that although the overall incidence of cervical cancer has fallen, its incidence amongst young women is rising. Young adults' rates of mental health problems more generally, and schizophrenia, stress-related illnesses and depression more specifically, have also attracted much attention in policy circles in recent years (Rogers and Pilgrim, 2010; Sellström et al., 2010; Foley et al., 2011).

Discussion Point

Why do you think that young adulthood is a stage of adulthood where we experience our best health and well-being?

Life Before Adulthood

This is the first of the two sections of this chapter that examines health and well-being in young adulthood from a life course perspective. You will now be very familiar with the arguments put forward from this perspective about the way in which health and well-being outcomes are cumulative throughout the life course. In line with these arguments, using the examples discussed in Chapters 2, 3 and 4, the influence of risks that can occur in pre-pregnancy and during pregnancy, childhood and adolescence on health and well-being at this life stage will be addressed. The aforementioned examples are summarised in Table 5.1. This summary is not definitive but has been compiled with the aim of using the findings presented so far in this book in order to illustrate the way in which risks to health and well-being prior to adulthood can potentially accumulate and impact on this life stage.

Table 5.1   The impact of pre-adulthood risks to health and well-being during young adulthood

Pre-pregnancy influences	Outcomes for health and well-being in young adulthood
Maternal pre-pregnancy weight below 50 kg	This can lead to low birth weight, which in turn can result in a range of adverse health outcomes in adulthood, such as cardiovascular diseases, hypertension and diabetes
Fetal exposures	
Low-quality maternal diet	Poor fetal growth and low birth weight that can result in cardiovascular diseases, hypertension, obesity and diabetes in adulthood
Obesity in pregnancy	Increases risk of abnormality
Risks associated with certain foods, such as uncooked meat, fish, eggs	Hydrocephalus (water on the brain), brain damage, epilepsy, deafness, blindness and growth problems
Maternal alcohol consumption	Physical and neurodevelopmental problems as a result of fetal abnormalities. Examples of these problems are facial deformities, physical and emotional developmental problems, memory and attention deficits, as well as cognitive and behavioural problems
Prenatal stress	As this can lead to low birth weight, the risks of cardiovascular diseases, hypertension and diabetes are increased. Exposure to maternal stress during intrauterine life may also increase the risk in young adulthood of a range of negative physical and mental health outcomes, such as metabolic dysfunction, immune dysfunction, hypothalamic-pituitary-adrenal endocrine dysregulation and cognitive (working memory) dysfunction

Fetal exposures	Outcomes for health and well-being in young adulthood
Maternal antenatal depression	Increased vulnerability to depression and abnormalities of the neuroendocrine systems in adulthood
Smoking and regular exposure to smoke-filled environments in pregnancy	Increased risk of psychiatric problems in young adulthood
Uncontrolled Type 1 or Type 2 diabetes	The effects of congenital malformation in adulthood

Childhood risks	
Birth trauma	The effects of irreversible brain, skeletal and organ damage that can have lifelong consequences for health and well-being. Traumatic birth experiences can also lead to childbirth-related post-traumatic stress disorder in mothers. Amongst the outcomes of such disorders is an inability to bond with the child that affects psychological health in adulthood
Maternal depression	Mental health problems as a result of the impact of maternal depression on a mother's parenting style. Maternal depression can also lead to a higher risk of infections in children up to the age of 4 years and this in turn can increase the risk of chronic diseases, such as cardiovascular disease, in adulthood
Childhood illnesses	Higher rates of cancer, lung disease, cardiovascular conditions and arthritis/rheumatism have been found in adults who suffered from certain illnesses in childhood. Some conditions, such as congenital heart defects (CHD), can lead to communication and social impairment. Ill health in childhood may also have socioeconomic consequences in adulthood
Early menarche	There is an association with menarche at the age of 12 or less with the risk of metabolic disease in early adulthood and breast cancer throughout adulthood
Undiagnosed mental health problems	Increased vulnerability to mental health problems. In addition, aggression in childhood that is not effectively treated is associated with problems in adulthood, such as anti-social personality disorders, alcohol and drug misuse, criminality and unemployment
Passive smoking	Respiratory diseases, asthma, leukaemia, lymphoma, lung cancer and brain tumours in adulthood
Smoking	Psychological problems, respiratory diseases, vascular disease and chronic obstructive pulmonary disease (COPD), as well as many forms of cancers. The latter include lung, upper aero-digestive tract (oral cavity, nasal cavity, nasal sinuses, pharynx, larynx and oesophagus), pancreas, stomach, liver, bladder, kidney, cervix, bowel and ovarian cancer, as well as myeloid leukaemia

(Continued)

Table 5.1 *(Continued)*

Childhood risks	Outcomes for health and well-being in young adulthood
Diet and nutrition	An inadequate diet in childhood that contains an excess of fat and sugar intake and not enough fruit, vegetables and high-fibre products can lead to many physical and mental health problems in adulthood. Examples of these are high cholesterol, cardiovascular diseases, diabetes, high blood pressure and depression
Overweight and obesity	Greater risk of developing sleep apnoea, muscularskeletal disease, diabetes, hypertension, heart disease, liver disease, pulmonary disease, some cancers, asthma and mental ill health. The life-threatening consequences some of these have for health and well-being can mean that there is a loss of health-related quality of life and a shortened lifespan
Being a bully	Those who are bullies in childhood are more likely to exhibit anti-social behavior in adulthood, as well as problems with maintaining stable relationships and long-term employment
Being bullied	Bullied children are at risk of substance abuse and of being victimised in young adulthood
Child abuse	Increased vulnerability to drug abuse, mental health problems, psychiatric disorders, offending and anti-social behaviour
Insecure parental attachments and ineffective parenting	Poorer mental health and emotional well-being, as well as developing a substance abuse problem and an unhealthy relationship with alcohol
Conflict between parents	Aggressive conflict in personal relationships
Risks in adolescence	
Chronic illnesses in adolescence	Emotional and developmental problems, serious medical conditions, ongoing anxiety, reduced employment prospects, secondary cancer or treatment-related cancer in later life, fertility issues that in turn affect well-being and life planning, higher risk of mortality
Poor mental health	Major depression, suicidal behaviour, alcoholism, anti-social personality disorders, drug misuse, as well as relationship problems, decreased employment opportunities, lower income, lower owner-occupation rates and increased probability of criminal activity
Anorexia nervosa and bulimia nervosa	Heart and gastrointestinal diseases, infertility, nerve damage and osteoporosis
Reduced physical activity rates	Leads to a reduction in average energy expenditure that can contribute to obesity. The outcomes of obesity in adolescence for health and well-being in young adulthood are outlined below

Risks in adolescence	Outcomes for health and well-being in young adulthood
Poor nutrition	Adolescents in this country generally have lower levels of vegetable and fruit consumption. This can increase their risks of cancer and coronary heart disease in later life
Overweight and obesity	Risk of developing sleep apnoea, high blood pressure (a major cause of strokes), high cholesterol levels, mental illness, heart disease, liver disease, cancer and diabetes as adults. In addition, there is evidence that obesity in adulthood leads to a loss in health-related quality of life
Inconsistent use of contraception and high number of sexual partners	Higher rates of sexually transmitted diseases and unplanned pregnancies. The former can lead to ectopic pregnancy, miscarriage, infertility and chronic illnesses (including some cancers) in later life. With reference to HIV, this can cause Acquired Immune Deficiency Syndrome (AIDS), which in turn can result in life-threatening infections and cancers. Abortion of an unplanned pregnancy in adolescence has been shown to lead to an increased risk of breast cancer, pelvic inflammatory disease, depression and the contraction of viral hepatitis in the longer term
Smoking	Smoking-related illnesses in later life. Whilst the main smoking-related illness is lung cancer, smoking does cause other cancers such as cancer of the upper aero-digestive tract (oral cavity, nasal cavity, nasal sinuses, pharynx, larynx and oesophagus), pancreas, stomach, liver, bladder, kidney, cervix, bowel, ovary and myeloid leukaemia. Other illnesses that are recognised as being related to smoking are respiratory, vascular and chronic obstructive pulmonary diseases (COPD)
Regular drug use	Serious and/or persistent offending and a drug use career
Binge drinking	Increased risk of psychological problems, the effects of irreversible brain damage, cognitive impairments, ischaemic heart disease, liver disease, infertility and development of an alcohol-related disorder and/or alcoholism
Poverty and deprivation	Poorer health and well-being in general, increased risks of cardiovascular disease, obesity and Type 2 diabetes in adulthood, as well as lower educational attainment, employment and socioeconomic status

Our discussions in this book so far have shown how health risks accumulate across the life course and that the number of risks to health and well-being from previous life stages increases quite dramatically at each new life stage. This point is clearly demonstrated in Table 5.1. Not only is it longer than the equivalent tables in Chapters 3 and 4 but it also shows that on entering adulthood an individual's health and well-being can be threatened by more events and influences from preceding life stages than when he or she entered adolescence. However, as we have seen in other chapters, these risks to health and well-being are mediated by a number of interacting variables. With reference to those experienced during adolescence, variables such as gender, personality, culture, the media, youth subcultures, ethnicity, religiosity, parental influences, poverty and social disadvantage can play an impact role. Furthermore, as discussed, some of these variables have 'protective effects' (Bryant et al., 2003: 363) and can counteract exposure to some risk factors. For instance, religiosity can have protective qualities in relation to mental distress, substance use and risk-taking sexual activity. Similarly, the quality of parenting and family relations can reduce some of the worse effects of poverty and social disadvantage in adolescence.

Although the information in Table 5.1 makes a significant contribution to our understanding of health and well-being in young adulthood from a life course perspective, it does not account for the effects of any interacting variables on the risks identified within it. An exploration of young adulthood from a life course perspective is also incomplete without considering the evidence about those factors that are most likely to compromise health and well-being during this life stage and their implications for middle and older age. It is to this evidence that we now turn.

Risks to Health and Well-Being During Young Adulthood

The decline in risk-taking behaviours that occurs during late adolescence continues into the first few years of young adulthood; the evidence shows that risk taking is more common up until our mid twenties than in later young adulthood. Indeed, it is argued that the way in which chlamydia and HIV mortality rates level off during the late twenties and thirties is due in part to less risk-taking behaviour after the age of 25. As we progress through our twenties and thirties there are other priorities in our lives, such as relationships, family life and employment. This reprioritisation is reflected in the risks to health and well-being in young adulthood that have been identified in the literature and are discussed in the rest of this section. We will start with findings about typical risk-taking behaviour, such as substance abuse, and demonstrate how these tend to be more the preserve of those in early adulthood. The discussions then move on to various other aspects of young adulthood and how these impact on health and well-being both at this life stage and in later life.

ACTIVITY 5.1

The grid set out below uses the same format as that in Table 5.1. When reading through this section of the chapter, try to identify any risks that are likely to affect health and well-being in midlife and make a note of them on the grid. This activity is designed to help you continue to develop your ability to interpret the findings about health and well-being at a particular life stage from a life course perspective.

Risks in young adulthood	Outcomes for health and well-being in midlife

Substance Abuse

As in Chapter 4, we will focus on smoking, drinking and use of recreational drugs in relation to substance use. Whilst the patterns in young adults' use of each of these substances and the possible risks to health and well-being are discussed below, several more general trends in substance use amongst young adults emerge from the studies that have been carried out. These include the way in which use of each of these substances tends to peak during the early years of young adulthood and then decrease, often rapidly. In addition, their use is normally positively associated (such as smoking and unsafe drinking) and when such association occurs the threat to health and well-being increases considerably (Hart et al., 2010; Smith and Krishnan-Sarin, 2010). Although the possible risks to health and well-being identified in the discussions mainly focus on the physiological effects of the use of each substance on physical and mental well-being, the literature shows that there are also many social consequences. Examples of these are relationship breakdown and unemployment that in turn impact on health and well-being (Collins et al., 2007; Littlefield and Sher, 2010; Nunes, 2010).

Smoking

Until recently, young adults in Western countries had the highest rates of smoking within any given population. However, since 2009, the smoking rates in the United Kingdom have declined (Smith and Krishnan-Sarin, 2010; Office for National Statistics, 2011b). Those young adults who do smoke are at risk of developing nicotine dependence, the essential features of which are withdrawal and tolerance symptoms. The former include 'depressed mood, insomnia, irritability, anxiety, difficulty concentrating, restlessness and increased appetite and cravings for tobacco/nicotine' (Smith and Krishnan-Sarin, 2010: 214). Tolerance refers to desensitisation to the effects of nicotine, which reduces the neurochemical reward of nicotine and hence increases frequency of nicotine use. In addition, because considerable neurodevelopment occurs in young adulthood, studies show that nicotine use in young adulthood can have a lasting neurological impact. The number of cigarettes smoked in young adulthood have also been found to predict a range of psychiatric disorders, such as schizophrenia and substance abuse disorder (Sørensen et al., 2011). Furthermore, smoking is recognised as the single greatest cause of preventable illness and early death in adulthood (Office for National Statistics, 2011b). As we saw in Chapter 4, it can lead to serious diseases, such as respiratory disease, vascular disease and chronic obstructive pulmonary disease (COPD). It is also a major cause of lung cancer and many other types of cancers (see p. 71).

Alcohol Consumption

Whilst excessive alcohol consumption is the current norm in early adulthood, consumption of alcohol becomes more moderate in the middle and later phases of this life stage (Seaman and Ikegwuonu, 2010). Unfortunately, those who do engage in frequent heavy episodic drinking in early adulthood have been found to experience the same sort of adverse outcomes for health and well-being as adolescents who binge drink (see Chapter 4). They also have higher rates of alcohol dependence and abuse in their mid to late thirties (Sloan et al., 2011). Alcohol dependence and alcohol abuse or harmful use can cause substantial morbidity and mortality. Continued heavy alcohol use also hastens the onset of heart disease, stroke, cancers and liver cirrhosis by affecting the cardiovascular, gastrointestinal and immune systems. In addition, heavy drinking can result in amnesia, temporary cognitive deficits, sleep problems, peripheral neuropathy, gastrointestinal problems and a decrease in bone density and production of blood cells (Schuckit, 2009).

Recreational Drug Use

Many young adults will use recreational drugs occasionally and view it as part of normal socialising. Their highest rates of usage are in their early twenties. After this point in their lives most revert to occasional use or cease altogether. Those who continue to use recreational drugs on a regular basis in their late twenties and thirties are more likely to become drug dependent. Whilst occasional use in young adulthood is unlikely to cause long-term harm, when such use develops into dependence it can seriously threaten health and well-being. The effects vary in accordance with the type of drug. For instance, cocaine can lead to impaired judgement, paranoia, transient psychosis, depression, suicidal ideation and cardiovascular events. Opiods can cause apathy, respiratory depression and sudden death from respiratory arrest. There are also co-occurring psychiatric disorders that are associated with drug abuse more generally. Examples are major depression, bipolar disorder, anxiety disorders and attention deficit hyperactivity disorder (ADHD). In the longer term, whatever drug they take, drug abusers have lower incomes, greater welfare dependence and unemployment and lower relationship and life satisfaction. They are also at an increased risk of a drug use career, serious and/or persistent offending, as well as premature, often drug-related and violent death in middle adulthood (Fergusson and Boden, 2008; Nunes, 2010; Järvinen and Ravn, 2011: Nyhlén et al., 2011).

Overweight and Obesity

Starting out on adult life being overweight means increased risks of sleep apnoea, high blood pressure (a major cause of strokes), high cholesterol levels, hearing loss, mental illness and many chronic diseases that can potentially shorten the lifespan. Examples of these chronic diseases are heart disease, liver disease, cancers and diabetes. Such risks increase if obesity continues throughout young adulthood. There is also evidence that health-related quality of life is adversely affected by obesity in young adulthood (*Foresight Report*, 2007; Patton et al., 2011).

Some studies have focused specifically on the outcomes of being overweight or obese in young adulthood for health in later life, irrespective of when these problems started. A very recent study has found that having a high **Body Mass Index (BMI)** at the ages of 23 and 33 is associated with worse hearing at age 45 (Ecob et al., 2011). Other studies have looked at decreases in life expectancy for both males and females. As mentioned previously, a person is considered obese if they have a BMI of 30 or more. This study found that in the United Kingdom, a 30-year-old non-smoking man with a BMI of 35 is projected to lose five years of life compared to a similar person with a BMI of 24. The analogous result for women is a loss of two years. These findings match those in other Western countries. Other gender differences that have been identified include findings that obese young men experience increased morbidity, including fatal morbidity, from many diseases throughout life (Zimmerman et al., 2011). With reference to obese female young adults, studies have shown that they are less likely to marry and have poorer employment opportunities and lower incomes than other women (Kuh et al., 2005).

Intimate Relationships

The research about intimate relationships in young adulthood has been criticised for ignoring the increasing diversity of these relationships, for example same sex unions. Therefore, this literature does not provide a full understanding of the effects of intimate relationships on health and well-being in young adulthood and in subsequent life stages. However, it does highlight some important issues, mainly around the changing nature of these relationships.

Marriage has become increasingly optional as a context for intimate partnerships and the median age of marriage has risen significantly in recent decades. Consequently, most young adults will experience romantic relationships and non-relationship sexual partnering before they get married. Several implications of this change in intimate relationship formation for health and well-being have been identified. One of the main implications is the increased risk of sexually transmitted infections and unplanned pregnancies. The adverse effects of both of these were explained in Chapter 4 (see pp. 69–70). Another consequence of marital delay is that the majority of young adults have lived with a romantic partner by their mid twenties and 'cohabitation is now the modal pathway to marriage' (Sassler, 2010: 5). Cohabitation results in a relatively unstable living arrangement and studies show that cohabiting couples report higher levels of discord and lower levels of subjective well-being than married couples. Although those who are married are comparatively happier in their intimate relationships, their levels of marital satisfaction do vary considerably throughout this life stage. For instance, the happiest married couples are those without children and less than five years into their relationship (Sassler, 2010; Economic and Social Research Council, 2011).

Where marriage leads to marital satisfaction, it generally encourages individuals (especially men) to engage in healthier lifestyles, as well as improving life satisfaction and health and well-being. Studies have shown that heart failure and cancer survival rates are higher for married patients. Married men also tend to have lower morbidity and mortality rates (Fincham and Beach, 2010; Gerward et al., 2010; Kravdal and Syse, 2011). Nonetheless, the benefits of marriage for health and well-being are not consistent over the life course; prolonged marital conflict can lead to poorer mental and physical health, including 'increased depressive symptoms and functional impairment ... and the onset of several psychiatric disorders ... mood, anxiety and substance abuse disorders' (Fincham and Beach, 2010: 633).

Another change in intimate relationships is that there are now more relationship dissolutions and divorces. Indeed, 'divorce has replaced death as the most frequent end point of marriage' (Fincham and Beach, 2010: 632). This change in intimate relationships increases the probability that a sizeable share of young adults do not live with a partner at some point during this life stage. The preoccupation in young adulthood with forming romantic relationships and selecting mates for the long term exacerbates the anxieties of those who find themselves without a partner at this life stage. In addition, those who experience dissolution of their intimate relationships (marital and non-marital) have more symptoms of depression and anxiety and higher rates of substance abuse. They are also at greater risk of more physical and mental health problems, both during young adulthood and in later life, and of overall mortality (Amato, 2010; Bracke et al., 2010). A further consequence of both marital and non-marital relationship dissolution is that many individuals will re-enter the partner market with prior cohabiting or marital experience. New intimate relationships therefore often involve the formation of remarried families and stepfamilies. These bring their own challenges and stressors in that they are built on existing foundations of partnership, parenthood and extended kin relations. This is reflected in the lower levels of well-being associated with remarriages at any stage in life and shorter duration of second and subsequent marriages compared with first marriages (Sassler, 2010; Sweeney, 2010).

ACTIVITY 5.2

How are you doing with your grid? Here are some suggestions about points that you could have included so far for you to check out.

Risks in young adulthood	Outcomes for health and well-being in midlife
Smoking	Neurological damage, a range of psychiatric disorders (for example, schizophrenia and substance abuse disorder), respiratory disease, vascular disease and chronic obstructive pulmonary disease (COPD), lung and many other types of cancers
Excessive alcohol consumption	Higher rates of alcohol dependence and abuse, mortality, heart disease, stroke, cancers, and liver cirrhosis, amnesia, peripheral neuropathy, gastrointestinal problems and decreased bone density, blood cell production, relationship breakdown and unemployment
Recreational drug use	Psychiatric disorders, lower income, welfare dependence, unemployment, lower life satisfaction, increased risk of a drug use career, serious and/or persistent offending, relationship breakdown and unemployment, drug-related and violent death
Overweight and obesity	High blood pressure (a major cause of strokes), high cholesterol levels, hearing loss, mental illness, as well as chronic diseases (such as heart disease and diabetes) and some cancers that can potentially shorten the lifespan
Non-relationship sexual partnering	Legacies of sexually transmitted infections and unplanned pregnancies
Prolonged marital/ relationship conflict	Poorer mental and physical health, including depression, psychiatric disorders, mood, anxiety and substance abuse disorders
Dissolution of intimate relationships	Physical and mental health problems, overall lower level of well-being associated with formation of new intimate relationships

Parenthood

The transformative process of parenthood is most likely to take place during young adulthood (Beckett, 2009). As Figure 5.1 shows, most people have their first child between the ages of 20 and 39.

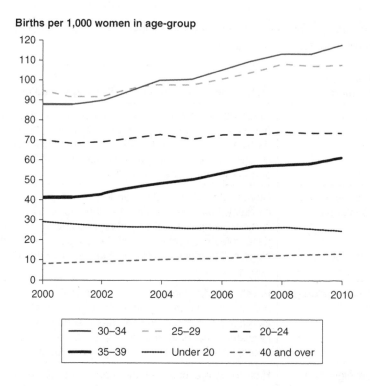

Births per 1,000 women in age-group

30–34	
25–29	
20–24	
35–39	
Under 20	
40 and over	

Figure 5.1   Age-specific fertility rates, England and Wales, 2000–10

Source: Office for National Statistics (2011a).

Central to this transformative process is pregnancy and childbirth. Although the risks of pregnancy and childbirth are much lower in Western countries than in many other parts of the world and have considerably reduced in recent decades, they still present a significant threat to health and well-being at this life stage (World Health Organization et al., 2010). Risks associated with pregnancy are **venous thrombosis** (or blood clot), back pain, headaches, sleeplessness, feeling tired, hypertension, depression, incontinence, **gestational diabetes** and **pre-eclampsia**. Some of these are more serious than others. For instance, women with gestational diabetes during their pregnancy have a higher incidence of Type 2 diabetes in later life. Indeed, some studies have shown that women with a history of gestational diabetes are at a higher risk of developing Type 2 diabetes within five years of delivery (Gunderson et al., 2011). If pre-eclampsia is left untreated, it can result in a stroke, impaired kidney and liver function, blood-clotting problems, fluid on the lungs, seizures and, on rare occasions, the mother's death. Pre-eclampsia has also been linked to 'higher risk of coronary heart disease incidence and mortality' (Rich-Edwards, 2002: 33) long after childbearing. Maternal characteristics that increase the risk of pre-eclampsia include being over 35, being overweight and having high blood pressure before becoming pregnant. Other risks in pregnancy, such as incontinence and venous thrombosis, may require treatment after pregnancy and hence have longer-term implications for health and well-being.

With reference to childbirth itself, the most frequent complications in childbirth or the postpartum period are severe bleeding, infections, obstructed labour, depression and **puerperal psychoses**. Without effective medical intervention, postpartum bleeding and obstructed labour can be fatal. Between 10 and 15 per cent of women experience postnatal depression. Since the 1990s, it has been acknowledged that this condition also affects men after their wives or partners have given birth. Advances in the treatment of depression and puerperal psychoses mean that both conditions can usually be resolved within a few weeks. However, a small minority of women who suffer a puerperal episode do go on to experience similar episodes in later life. Although these can be related to the menstrual cycle and/or the birth of other children, there are cases where such episodes are completely unrelated to childbearing (Rich-Edwards, 2002; Robson and Waugh, 2008; Lee, 2010).

The excitement and trauma of pregnancy and childbirth is inevitably followed by the responsibility of caring for a newborn baby 24 hours a day. Many mothers find this emotionally and physically exhausting. The exhaustion combined with sleep deprivation and changes in hormone levels can result in them feeling stressed and overwhelmed. Nonetheless, not all aspects of this role have negative consequences for health and well-being; studies have shown that if mothers breastfeed, it increases the likelihood that they use up body fat deposited during pregnancy. Moreover, the benefits of breastfeeding have also been found to extend to the mothers' longer-term health in that they can reduce the likelihood of developing some forms of ovarian cancer and premenopausal breast cancer (Kelly and Watt, 2005; Dyson et al., 2007).

The birth of a first child in young adulthood is simultaneously a major life transition. Like all other such transitions, parenthood triggers shifts in well-being. It is shaped by a variety of contextual features that means that for some it is an important source of well-being whilst for others it is a profound stressor. One such contextual feature is timing; early transitions into parenthood have been associated with truncated educational and work opportunities as well as increased depression and marital instability. Age is also influential; women experience the greatest increases in well-being if they have their first child between the ages of 23 and 30. Where couples are cohabiting as opposed to married, studies have shown that becoming a parent leads to a decline in psychological well-being. Given the trend towards childlessness in recent decades, it is equally important to consider the effects of not transitioning into parenthood at this life stage. Although childless young adults report better well-being than parents, this is often not the case for those whose fertility intentions were thwarted (McMahon, 2010; Umberson et al., 2010).

The effects of the transition into parenthood at this life stage can persist throughout the life course in that it impacts on middle and older age. For instance, early or later (after the age of 30) transition to parenthood has been linked to increased risks of breast cancer, poorer self-rated health in midlife and more depression in older life.

Depressive symptoms are notably higher in later life for those whose transition into parenthood was earlier or later than their expectations about the timing of this transition in their lives. In relation to childlessness, although childless women have higher breast cancer rates throughout adulthood, there is some evidence that the childless have less depression than parents during their forties and fifties (see Chapter 6) and are less prone to long-term, cumulative weight gain. With respect to old age, childlessness has been found to be associated with decreased health and well-being for unmarried men and formerly married men only; childless older women seem to enjoy less depression and more social activity than parents (Rich-Edwards, 2002; Umberson et al., 2010; Carlson, 2011).

Once the transition into parenthood has been made, how does parenthood itself impact on the health and well-being of young adults? The evidence is confusing; there are those who argue that 'children do not make you less happy; it's just that children don't make you *more* happy' (Senior, 2010: 15). However, some groups of parents, particularly parents of young children, those on a low income, single parents and stepmothers, find parenthood very stressful. Reasons given include the demands and constraints that young children place on parents' time, work–family conflict and, where there are two parents, the tensions that they cause between them. Furthermore, parenthood in general invariably reduces marital satisfaction and has its worst effects on couples who became parents before marriage. Such stress and relationship strain undermines physical and psychological well-being and has in turn been associated with early onset hypertension for mothers. Hypertension in young adulthood is positively associated in later life with cardiovascular disease and cardiovascular disease mortality (McCarron et al., 2000). The aforementioned stresses and strains can also lead to an increase in the incidence of certain mental health problems and a decrease in participation in physical activities for both parents (Kahneman et al., 2004; Marshall and Tracy, 2009; Umberson et al., 2010; Sjögren et al., 2011). With reference to mental health problems, the onset of schizophrenia in parenthood has been attributed to the fact that the nature of the role expectations of parenthood is incompatible with this illness. Therefore, if hitherto undiagnosed, schizophrenia becomes more apparent with parenthood (Rogers and Pilgrim, 2010).

Employment

Although lack of employment in young adulthood has been found to lead to depression, self-harm, alcohol-related disorders and drug abuse, it is argued that it is impossible to clarify whether economic inactivity causes mental health problems or if having mental problems leads to economic inactivity (Sellström et al., 2010). Other ways in which lack of employment is a risk to health and well-being about which there is more clarity include the link between unemployment and poorer eating habits. Studies have shown that unemployment is associated with reduced consumption of fruits and vegetables and increased consumption of 'unhealthy' foods such as snacks and fast food (Dave and Kelly, 2012). When in employment, young adults who work long hours (more than 48 hours per week) tend to have problems with sleeping. In the short term these can cause memory and cognitive impairment, and relationship stress, as well as increase the risk of having driving accidents and sustaining an occupational injury. In the longer term, there are many clinical consequences of untreated sleep problems, for example high blood pressure, heart attack, stroke, Type 2 diabetes, obesity and psychiatric problems (Spiegel et al., 1999; Economic and Social Research Council, 2011).

Mental Health

The discussions in this section so far have shown that there are several identifiable sources of threats to mental health in young adulthood, such as relationship, parenting and employment issues. Indeed, as we saw in the previous section, the incidence of mental health problems amongst young adults is in fact increasing and the most notable increases are in the incidence of schizophrenia, stress-related illnesses and depression. Studies have found that many young adults also experience a co-occurrence of their mental health problems with other medical illnesses. For example, depression and substance abuse often co-occur. In addition, depression has been found to be related to body weight variability and migraine as well as reduced chances of conceiving with *in vitro* fertilisation among young adults (Rich-Edwards, 2002; Suvisaari et al., 2009; Zarate, 2010).

There are some mental health problems that are more common early on in young adulthood than later on at this life stage. These include **obsessive compulsive disorder (OCD)** and eating disorders. Moreover, mental health problems which have their origins in the first few years of this life stage pose greater risks to health and well-being in the longer term. Along with adolescence, the early part of young adulthood is a time in the life course when mental health problems are most likely to develop (McCrone et al., 2008; Crow, 2010). However, effective treatment is typically not initiated until a number of years later. There is increasing evidence that this lack of intervention can result in more severe and persistent symptoms of primary disorders and the development of secondary disorders and hence accumulation of mental health problems in later life (McGorry et al., 2011). Furthermore, whether it is undetected or not, having a psychiatric disorder in your early twenties or at any point during young adulthood has been found to be associated with relationship breakdown, reduced workforce participation, lower income and lower economic living standards (Suvisaari et al., 2009; Gibb et al., 2010).

Long-Term Illnesses

The way that the incidence of chronic illnesses amongst adolescents has increased was discussed in Chapter 4. There are now more young adults with chronic illnesses. Let us use the examples of diabetes and cancer once more in order to illustrate some of the implications of long-term illnesses for health and well-being at this life stage. With reference to diabetes, in addition to the psychological and medical complications, those with Type 1 and Type 2 diabetes are at a higher risk of mortality until they are 34. After this point, mortality rates then start to decrease as age increases. Turning to cancer, increasing cancer diagnoses in adolescence and young adulthood mean that there are now more young adults who have experienced cancer as adolescents and more young adults with cancer. Both these groups are at risk of secondary cancer or treatment-related cancer, ongoing anxiety, emotional problems and loss of fertility during young adulthood. In addition, research has shown that they can experience reduced employment prospects (particularly females), employment related **discrimination** and problems obtaining mortgages and insurance (Grinyer, 2007, 2009; Torp et al., 2012).

More generally, young adults who have any form of physical and psychological long-term illness face similar problems with regard to employment. A recent study found that experiencing illnesses in young adulthood represents 'a greater risk of labour market exclusion compared to later in life' (van der Wel, 2011: 1097), either because those concerned find it much harder to gain employment or, if employed, are more likely to become unemployed. Hence it is argued that from a life course perspective, young adulthood may be regarded as a social equivalent to the biological 'critical period'. This is because 'it is a phase in life in which risk exposure could potentially affect an individual's future health, social position, material resources and working life prospects in profound ways' (van der Wel, 2011: 1097) (Bartley et al., 1997; van der Wel, 2011).

ACTIVITY 5.3

Finished your grid? Now compare the risks that are likely to affect health and well-being in young adulthood that you have identified with those in Table 6.1 in Chapter 6. Are there any differences? If so, why do you think that these differences exist?

Influences on the Risks to Health and Well-Being During Young Adulthood

In Chapter 1, we saw how the life course perspective on health and well-being not only emphasises the need to understand how the outcomes of risks to health and well-being accumulate throughout the life course but also the need to consider the many influences on our health and well-being at each life stage. The above discussions of the risks to health and well-being during young adulthood made reference either directly or indirectly to factors that shape their outcomes. For instance, there was evidence that gender plays a role in the effects of obesity on health and well-being. Similarly, cultural and social factors are clearly influential on the decrease in smoking rates amongst young adults and the changes in the timing of marriage and parenthood in their lives that were discussed. As at other life stages, the risks to health and well-being in young adulthood interact not only with themselves but also with these sorts of factors and the legacies of their role in previous life stages. When considering the role of previous and current influences on health and well-being during young adulthood it is also important to acknowledge the way in which positive influences can offset negative ones, and vice versa, in the way that they affect the accumulation of health outcomes from conception through to infancy, childhood, adolescence, adulthood and old age. With reference to previous influences, breastfeeding has been found to provide protection from adverse health outcomes in adulthood, for example diabetes and coronary heart disease (see Chapter 3). Personality characteristics, such as being able to take responsibility for your actions rather than being constantly shaped by the behaviours of others, self-understanding and emotional resilience have also been shown to counteract some of the negative influences on psychological well-being in young adulthood (Gralinski-Bakker et al., 2005; Burns at al., 2010).

ACTIVITY 5.4

The following are examples of the complexity of the interactions between different factors that play a role in young adults' health and well-being as presented in the findings in two different studies. See which ones you can identify in each statement. There are some ideas to help you at the end of the chapter.

- The happiest relationships are those less than five years in duration, between two people educated to degree level, who have no children and where the man is employed
- Childless couples are happiest with their relationships and those with preschool children are least happy, although happiness increases with the age of the youngest child
- Among men, being out of employment is associated with lower levels of happiness in their relationships with their partner. Income seems to be unrelated to relationship happiness among men, and is only mildly important for women
- Problems getting to sleep on three or more nights a week are particularly high under age 25, then decline slightly for men with age but increase with age for women

Adapted from Economic and Social Research Council (2011)

Generally, childless young adults report better well-being than parents, although childlessness in young adulthood has been shown to be stressful in the context of thwarted fertility intentions, especially for women with low incomes

Adapted from Umberson et al. (2010)

The literature on young adulthood provides more examples of the aforementioned influences on health and well-being at this life stage as well as examples of many others. In order to continue our exploration of the life course perspective in relation to young adulthood and assess the relative importance of this life stage in terms of health and well-being, we need to consider the role of these influences. The main influences identified are discussed below.

Cultural Influences

Several studies have addressed the role of cultural influences on substance use in young adulthood. Let us start with those that have focused on alcohol use. Levels of alcohol consumption in early adulthood in the United Kingdom are significantly higher than in many other European countries (Plant et al., 2010). Studies have attributed this to various cultural influences within this country. One is the change in young adults' socialising that has 'increasingly developed a culture that reinforces the need for drinking to participate and belong' (Seaman and Ikegwuonu, 2010: 3). This results in today's young adults finding it difficult to imagine alternatives to the excessive drinking that supports group socialising. The media and pricing have been found to be influential, too. With reference to the former, excessive alcohol consumption by young adults has been linked to the way in which the media used by young people commonly presents drinking alcohol as normal and unproblematic, without focusing on the negative consequences. Low-price alcohol has also been blamed as pricing has been found to override young adults' perceptions of health or risk in decision-making about alcohol consumption (Seaman and Ikegwuonu, 2010; Atkinson et al., 2011).

Nonetheless, such findings need to be considered alongside the evidence that there are many counterinfluences on alcohol consumption and the use of other substances in young adulthood that interact in complex ways. For instance, religiosity provides a protective effect against binge drinking, marijuana use and cigarette smoking but not for sexual minorities (Rostosky et al., 2007). Smoking rates vary considerably between young adults in different ethnic groups and between men and women within those groups; Bangladeshi and Irish men are more likely to smoke than the general male population, whereas Indian men are less likely to smoke. In comparison, Black African, South Asian and Chinese women are less likely to smoke than the rest of the female population (Department of Health, 2007). Such conflicting evidence makes drawing firm conclusions about cultural influences on substance use in young adulthood problematic.

Other cultural norms that are particularly influential on health and well-being at this life stage are those around male and female employment. The increase in women's participation in the labour market throughout their working lives means that when a child is born to a couple in a relationship, both parents usually work (Larkin, 2011a). This trend has been associated with role overload that in turn increases partnership dissatisfaction. The latter is often compounded by the fact that men's housework contribution is still much lower than that of their female partners (Gatrell, 2008; Green, 2010).

The economy

It is impossible to talk about cultural influences on health and well-being in young adulthood without considering the role of the economy. The current economic climate means that unemployment rates are highest amongst those under 25 (Economic and Social Research Council, 2011). In addition to the adverse effects of unemployment on health and well-being described above, the economic and employment uncertainty has led to higher burnout levels at this life stage and increased both the incidence of mental health disorders and the rate of suicide (Norlund et al., 2010; Royal College of Psychiatrists, 2010; Sellström et al., 2010).

The average age of homeownership has now risen to 31 and many argue that economic factors have also contributed significantly to this. One of the consequences of this rise is that more young adults have to live with their parents, which inevitably leads to a lack of independence and in turn has implications on the achievement of a full transition into adulthood (Clapham et al., 2010; Graham, 2010; Rugg, 2010).

Poverty and Social Disadvantage

In each chapter in this book so far we have seen how poverty and social disadvantage are key influences on health and well-being. There is also a wealth of evidence about how they affect young adulthood. The health of children from families with lower incomes erodes faster with age. Even after adjusting for health-related behaviour and improvements in their social circumstances in young adulthood, studies show that those who have grown up in a low-income family are at a greater risk of worse health during this life stage than those who grew up in families with a higher socioeconomic status (Kuh and Wadsworth, 1993; Palloni et al., 2009; Tucker-Seeley et al., 2011). In addition, this group of young adults are more likely to have had an accelerated transition into young adulthood because they have fewer economic and family resources. As a result, they face the stresses of adult life, such as work and parenthood, much earlier than those from more middle-class backgrounds (Green, 2010).

Whatever an individual's socioeconomic background prior to young adulthood, living in a socially disadvantaged neighbourhood and experiencing poverty at this life stage are linked to poorer physical and mental health both at this life stage and in later life (Johnson et al., 2012). Examples include higher rates of cardiovascular disease, obesity, Type 2 diabetes and stress (Umberson et al., 2010; Beauchamp et al., 2011; Marmot Review Team, 2011). Poverty and social disadvantage are also associated with poorer health-related behaviours, such as higher smoking and substance abuse rates, harmful alcohol consumption and lower rates of physical activity (Rayner et al., 2010; Boone-Heinonen et al., 2011; Giskes et al., 2011; Office for National Statistics, 2011b). However, recent evidence points to increases in substance abuse amongst young adults in higher socioeconomic groups (Humensky, 2010). Other consequences of poverty and social disadvantage in young adulthood are increased family conflict and family instability, poorer education, reduced employment and earnings prospects and higher offending rates (Bradshaw et al., 2006; Fincham and Beach, 2010; Spijkers et al., 2011; van der Wel, 2011).

Gender

The extent to which gender influences heath and well-being varies throughout young adulthood. Women's fertility declines significantly between 35 and 40, whereas for men there is no equivalent dramatic decline in reproductive function (Green, 2010). Up until the age of 25, the prevalence of eating disorders such as anorexia nervosa and bulimia nervosa is much higher amongst females. Men are more likely to have alcohol use disorders and die at this early stage of young adulthood than women, mainly because of car accidents and suicide (Bendelow, 2009; Zarate, 2010). With the exception of deaths from diabetes (these are higher for women between the ages of 15 and 34, see Chapter 4), after the age of 25 mortality statistics among men and women level off. Differences in their risk-taking behaviour such as smoking are reduced (Office for National Statistics, 2011b). As women aged 22 to 29 have now closed the gender pay gap and gender pay differentials only start to emerge around the age of 35, the effect of gender differences in income on health in young adulthood is not as significant as in other life stages (see Chapter 7) (Darlington et al., 2011). However, because they combine domestic and family duties with paid work to a far greater degree than men, studies have shown that women have a higher level of burnout than men, with the most pronounced difference being in the age group 35 to 44 (Norlund et al., 2010).

Discussion Point

To what extent do you think that the concept of 'sub-phases of young adulthood' is relevant to a life course analysis of health and well-being in young adulthood?

Reducing the Risks to Health and Well-Being During Young Adulthood

The problems of obtaining information about health and well-being in young adulthood as a separate life stage in adulthood were referred to in the Introduction to this chapter. As explained, these problems arise because of the infrequency of the distinction made between young and middle adulthood in the relevant literature. The same problems arise when analysing policy initiatives with a view to ascertaining how the risks to health and well-being during young adulthood are being addressed.

Most of the initiatives that have been introduced that are relevant to the health and well-being of young adults are directed at adults in general (Her Majesty's Treasury, 2004; Friedli, 2009; Atkinson et al., 2011). Those that do address the health and well-being of young adults specifically tend to focus on issues associated with childbirth, such as reducing maternal mortality and postnatal depression (National Institute for Health and Clinical Excellence, 2007a; McColl, 2010; WHO, World Bank, UNICEF and United Nations Population Fund, 2010). Interventions developed at national and international level, such as **exercise referral schemes,** healthy lifestyle and weight reduction schemes tend to focus on particular groups of adults as opposed to young adults, for example women from lower socioeconomic groups and those with chronic diseases (Schmidt et al., 2008; Claassen et al., 2010; Gray et al., 2011).

As the discussions in this chapter have shown, there are a number of threats to the health and well-being of adults in their twenties and thirties and some of these (the most notable examples being the effects of economic and employment uncertainty) are likely to increase. This suggests that there is a need for further research and attention to be focused on young adulthood as a life stage in itself in order to address effectively health and well-being across the life course.

Conclusions

This chapter has shown that health and well-being in young adulthood is not only shaped by events and influences in the preceding life stages but also by a range of factors. These can vary throughout this life stage; for instance, substance abuse is more likely to occur during the early part of this life stage. Furthermore, all the risks to health and well-being in young adulthood that were identified are shaped and modified by other variables to a greater or lesser extent.

At the end of Chapters 2, 3 and 4 in this book we returned to the question of whether the information presented supports Graham's view that pregnancy, childhood and adolescence are 'an unparalleled time during which external influences, both good and bad, can influence an individual's health and well-being across their whole life' (Graham, 2009: 26). Although it is not possible to examine this statement empirically, the literature and research that has been reviewed so far enables some conclusions to be drawn. The evidence that good and bad external influences in pregnancy, childhood and adolescence *do* shape many aspects of health and well-being across the whole of an individual's life course is unequivocal. However, other influences such as personality, genetic characteristics and gender should not be ignored. Moreover, as demonstrated in this chapter, there is plenty of evidence that 'external influences, both good and bad' in young adulthood are also highly important in shaping health and well-being in the years that follow. In addition, much of what has been presented in the chapters up to this point in the book shows that risks to health and well-being accumulate right across the life course. Further assessment of Graham's claims about the 'unparalleled' significance of pregnancy, childhood and adolescence is therefore required in relation to the life stages that follow young adulthood.

Summary

- Although there are changes in health and well-being across young adulthood, it is one of the healthiest times of life and overall the healthiest stage of adulthood; mortality rates are typically very low and people at this life stage are less affected by naturally occurring diseases and disabilities than older age groups
- Health issues amongst young adults that are causes for concern include increases in the rates of diabetes, obesity and mental health problems (schizophrenia, stress-related illnesses and depression more specifically) for both sexes, and the incidence of cervical cancer amongst young women
- From a life course perspective, on entering adulthood an individual's health and well-being can be threatened by more events and influences from preceding life stages than when he or she entered adolescence. However, these need to be considered alongside interacting variables that mediate any risks to health and well-being to which an individual has been exposed
- Identifiable risks to health and well-being during young adulthood include substance misuse, obesity, intimate relationships, parenthood, employment and mental health and long-term illnesses
- There is evidence that these risks to health and well-being during young adulthood are influenced by culture, the state of the economy, poverty, social disadvantage and gender
- Although there are a number of threats to the health and well-being of young adults, there are few initiatives that are relevant to their health and well-being specifically

Further Study

For a discussion of young adulthood as a life stage, see Chapter 5 in L. Green, *Understanding the Life Course: Sociological and Psychological Perspectives* (Cambridge: Polity Press, 2010). Although it is mainly based on American research, J.E. Grant and M.A. Potenza (eds), *Young Adult Mental Health* (New York: Oxford University Press, 2010), contains some useful chapters not only on mental health in young adulthood per se but also on relationships and substance abuse at this life stage. Books on lifespan development have informative sections on health and well-being in young adulthood. For example, K.S. Berger *The Developing Person through the Lifespan,* 8th edition (New York: Worth Publishers, 2011). If you are particularly interested in women's health, many of the chapters in D. Kuh and R. Hardy (eds), *A Life Course Approach to Women's Health* (Oxford: Oxford University Press, 2002), make significant contributions to our understanding of women's health and well-being in young adulthood.

Activity Comments

Suggestions about which factors interact in shaping young adults' health and well-being are in italics after each statement below:

- The happiest relationships are those less than five years in duration, between two people educated to degree level, who have no children and where the man is employed – *Length of relationship, level of education, absence of children, male employment*
- Childless couples are happiest with their relationships and those with preschool children are least happy, although happiness increases with the age of the youngest child – *Absence of children, age of children*
- Among men, being out of employment is associated with lower levels of happiness in their relationships with their partner. Income seems to be unrelated to relationship happiness among men, and is only mildly important for women – *Employment, gender (but not to any great extent)*
- Problems getting to sleep on three or more nights a week are particularly high under age 25, then decline slightly for men with age but increase with age for women – *Stage in young adulthood, gender*
- Generally, childless young adults report better well-being than parents, although childlessness in young adulthood has been shown to be stressful in the context of thwarted fertility intentions, especially for women with low incomes – *Childlessness, childbearing intentions, gender*

6

Health and Well-Being in Midlife

Overview

- Introduction
- Health and well-being in midlife
- Life before middle age
- Risks to health and well-being during midlife
- Negative *and* positive influences on the risks to health and well-being in midlife
- Prevention, prevention, prevention
- Conclusions
- Summary
- Further study
- Activity comments

Introduction

Although 'midlife' is movable chronologically because of changes in life expectancy and compulsory retirement age, it is currently used in relation to the period of our lives between 40 and 65. The terms 'second adulthood' and 'middle adulthood' are also used in the literature when referring to midlife. According to the data about health and well-being across the life course presented in Chapter 1, the percentage of both males and females in the population reporting 'good' general health continues its general decline throughout midlife. Although there are sharp increases in acute and chronic illnesses after the age of 45, mental distress decreases. As with young adulthood, obtaining detailed information about health and well-being in middle age is problematic because much of the research carried out to date does not distinguish between young and middle adulthood. It has also been referred to as 'the least researched age span' (Green, 2010: 149) and this is reflected in the length of some of the sections of this chapter when compared to those in the chapters on other life stages. Every attempt has been made to ensure that the material relevant to health and well-being in midlife that does exist is presented in this chapter. This material will also be used to reflect further (as in the other chapters in this book) on whether it is only the life stages of 'pregnancy, childhood and adolescence' that are 'unparalleled' in relation to the extent to which 'external influences, both good and bad, can influence an individual's health and well-being across their whole life' (Graham, 2009: 26) (Beckett, 2009; Green, 2010; Rees Jones et al., 2011).

The chapter will start by providing an overview of health and well-being during midlife. It will then move on to examine health and well-being at this life stage from a life course perspective. The first part of this examination will use findings from the discussions in the previous chapters about the effects of prenatal influences and exposure to risks during pregnancy, childhood, adolescence and young adulthood on health and well-being in midlife. During the second part, we will explore the potential risks to health and well-being during midlife as well as any implications for health and well-being in old age. Examples of the ways in which these risks can combine with risk factors from preceding life stages are also addressed in this section. This is followed by a discussion of both the negative and positive influences that shape health and well-being during midlife. As with the other chapters, the final section of this chapter analyses recent policy initiatives aimed at improving health and well-being in midlife.

Health and Well-Being in Midlife

This life stage has been divided up into various 'sub-phases', one of the most notable being the 'midlife transition' that is said to take place between 40 and 45 (Levinson, 1978). Features regarded as typical of midlife are often the outcome of historically specific cohort effects. For instance, changes in women's reproductive and working lives means that the concept of the **'empty nest syndrome'** seems increasingly redundant. Changes in women's reproductive lives include the way in which women are increasingly giving birth in their forties and, with the aid of reproductive technology, even in their fifties and sixties. Changes in women's working lives means that many mothers now work and are far less consumed by childcare and domestic life than mothers in previous generations (Office for National Statistics, 2011a). However, despite such 'sub-phases' and changes, there are some common themes in the literature about health and well-being in midlife.

This life stage is characterised by certain physical changes; hair becomes greyer and thinner, skin drier and less elastic, hearing, sight and smell decline, body fat increases and is more likely to be distributed around the stomach, buttocks and chin, there is a gradual reduction in metabolism, maximal heart rate, sex drive and physical performance as well as an increasing susceptibility to osteoporosis. As mentioned above, the incidence of chronic diseases increases during midlife. These include cancer, cardiovascular diseases, arthritis and high blood pressure. Using cancer as an example, whilst cancer rates do increase from the beginning of midlife, it is those over 50 who are at the greatest risk; over half of all cancers are diagnosed in 50- to 74-year-olds. Prostate cancer accounts for more than one in four cases diagnosed in males in this age group. Other common cancers for males are lung cancer and colorectal cancer. Over a third of cancer cases diagnosed in females aged 50 to 74 are breast cancers (Cancer Research UK, 2011). There is also a rise in disability rates after the age of 50 (Platt, 2011). Although there is some decline in speed of cognitive processing and working memory in middle age, improvements in other cognitive abilities (such as verbal memory, vocabulary, inductive reasoning and spatial orientation) as well as life experience and accumulated knowledge in general compensate for this. Women experience a continuing decline in fertility and the **menopause** with all its side effects and loss of fertility is most likely to occur around the middle of this life stage. Whilst men do not experience such dramatic declines in hormone levels or reproductive function, they do gradually produce less mobile and healthy sperm. Some critics claim that the female menopause has been increasingly medicalised. They also point to the way that the concept of the male menopause has been on and off the medical radar over a number of years and still remains an area of contention within the medical profession. Increasing life expectancy and the fact that there are significant differences in the rates at which middle-aged individuals age have similarly been used to challenge assumptions that midlife inevitably heralds the uncomfortable decline of old age (Hardy and Kuh, 2002; Hunt, 2005; Green, 2010).

The association between midlife and 'midlife crisis' is also debatable. Whilst midlife has been likened to a second adolescence because of the reappraisal of identity that occurs and adolescent-type behaviours that are exhibited, it is less turbulent than adolescence. Furthermore, there is a lack of agreement about the definition of the term 'midlife crisis' and it seems to be culturally relative. In addition, claims about the existence of a 'midlife crisis' remain unsubstantiated. Studies have identified emotional changes and losses that have to be addressed, for instance awareness of physical limitations, children leaving home, death of parents and fewer career options. However, they also show that midlife encompasses positive factors such as high levels of self-confidence and self-awareness, the benefits of accumulated knowledge, freedom to take on new challenges, grandparenthood, more disposable income and decreased relationship problems. Indeed, there is evidence that this is the life phase where we experience our highest levels of life satisfaction and our best mental health (Rogers and Pilgrim, 2003; Pilgrim 2007; Blanchflower and Oswald, 2008; de Ree and Alessie, 2011).

As middle-aged adults are prone to weight gain, there have been concerns in recent years about this group in relation to rising obesity levels. There has also been a strong emphasis on health screening and health prevention in midlife, for example cancer screening and blood pressure, weight and cholesterol monitoring (Minet Kinge and Morris, 2010; Lindvall et al., 2010; Emslie et al., 2011).

Life Before Middle Age

Our exploration of health and well-being in midlife from a life course perspective starts in this section by looking at how health and well-being at this life stage can be influenced by exposure to risks in preceding life stages. The effects of prenatal influences, together with risks to health and well-being that can occur during pregnancy, childhood, adolescence and young adulthood are summarised in Table 6.1 below. This summary is based on the reviews of the research and literature undertaken in Chapters 2 to 5 and is therefore only as comprehensive as the reviews themselves. Nonetheless, it provides tangible evidence of the cumulative nature of health and well-being outcomes.

Even though there are more threats to our health and well-being in midlife from previous life stages than any of the life stages discussed so far in this book, it is important to remember that these risks do not necessarily become reality. As explained in other chapters, the life course perspective recognises that such risks are shaped both positively and negatively by a range of interacting variables. Examples of these variables discussed in Chapter 5 in relation to risks to health and well-being in young adulthood were cultural and economic influences, poverty, social disadvantage and gender. Whilst some aspects of these variables increase the risk of certain threats to health and well-being, others counteract the effects of these threats. For instance, poverty and social disadvantage are generally associated with higher smoking rates for men and women, ethnicity can have 'protective effects' (Bryant et al., 2003: 363) for women, in that Black African, South Asian and Chinese women are less likely to smoke than the rest of the female population.

A full understanding of health and well-being in midlife from a life course perspective requires not only the exploration of risks and influences at previous life stages on health and well-being at this life stage, but also the exploration of factors that can potentially compromise health and well-being during midlife. We will explore these factors in the next section of this chapter.

Discussion Point

Look at Table 6.1 again. To what extent do you think that screening and preventative measures can reduce the risks to health and well-being in midlife?

Table 6.1   The impact of pre-midlife risks to health and well-being during middle adulthood

Pre-pregnancy influences	Outcomes for health and well-being in midlife
Maternal pre-pregnancy weight below 50 kg	This can lead to low birth weight, which in turn can result in a range of adverse health outcomes in adulthood, such as cardiovascular diseases, hypertension and diabetes
Fetal exposures	
Low-quality maternal diet	Poor fetal growth and low birth weight that can result in cardiovascular diseases, hypertension, obesity and diabetes and female breast cancer
Obesity in pregnancy	Increases risk of abnormality
Risks associated with certain foods such as uncooked meat, fish, eggs	Hydrocephalus (water on the brain), brain damage, epilepsy, deafness, blindness and growth problems
Maternal alcohol consumption	Physical and neurodevelopmental problems as a result of fetal abnormalities. Examples of these problems are facial deformities, physical and emotional developmental problems, memory and attention deficits, as well as cognitive and behavioural problems
Prenatal stress	As this can lead to low birth weight, the risks of cardiovascular diseases, hypertension and diabetes are increased
Maternal antenatal depression	Increased vulnerability to depression and abnormalities of the neuroendocrine systems in adulthood
Smoking and regular exposure to smoke-filled environments in pregnancy	Increased risk of heart attacks and strokes in midlife
Uncontrolled Type 1 or Type 2 diabetes	The effects of congenital malformation
Childhood risks	
Birth trauma	The effects of irreversible brain, skeletal and organ damage that can have lifelong consequences for health and well-being. Traumatic birth experiences can also lead to childbirth-related post-traumatic stress disorder in mothers. Amongst the outcomes of such disorders is an inability to bond with the child that affects psychological health in adulthood
Maternal depression	Mental health problems as a result of the impact of maternal depression on a mother's parenting style. Maternal depression can also lead to a higher risk of infections in children up to the age of four years and this in turn can increase the risk of chronic diseases in adulthood, such as cardiovascular disease

Childhood risks	Outcomes for health and well-being in midlife
Childhood illnesses	Higher rates of cancer, lung disease, arthritis, rheumatism and cardiovascular conditions have been found in adults who suffered from certain illnesses in childhood. Some conditions, such as congenital heart defects (CHD), can lead to communication and social impairment. Ill health in childhood may also have socioeconomic consequences in adulthood
Early menarche	There is an association with menarche at the age of 12 or less with an increased risk of breast cancer throughout adulthood
Undiagnosed mental health problems	Increased vulnerability to mental health problems. Aggression in childhood that is not effectively treated is also associated with problems in adulthood such as anti-social personality disorders, alcohol and drug misuse, criminality and unemployment
Passive smoking	Respiratory diseases, asthma, leukaemia, lymphoma, lung cancer and brain tumours in adulthood
Smoking	Psychological problems, respiratory diseases, vascular disease and chronic obstructive pulmonary disease (COPD), as well as many forms of cancers. The latter include lung, upper aero-digestive tract (oral cavity, nasal cavity, nasal sinuses, pharynx, larynx and oesophagus), pancreas, stomach, liver, bladder, kidney, cervix, bowel and ovarian cancer, as well as myeloid leukaemia
Diet and nutrition	An inadequate diet in childhood that contains an excess of fat and sugar intake and not enough fruit, vegetables and high-fibre products can lead to many physical and mental health problems in adulthood. Examples of these are high cholesterol, cardiovascular diseases, diabetes, high blood pressure and depression
Overweight and obesity	Greater risk of developing sleep apnoea, muscularskeletal disease, diabetes, hypertension, heart disease, liver disease, pulmonary disease, some cancers, asthma and mental ill health. The life-threatening consequences that some of these have for health and well-being can mean that there is a loss of health-related quality of life and a shortened lifespan
Being a bully	Those who are bullies in childhood are more likely to exhibit anti-social behavior in adulthood, as well as problems with maintaining stable relationships and long-term employment
Being bullied	Bullied children are at risk of being victimised in adulthood

(Continued)

Table 6.1 *(Continued)*

Childhood risks	Outcomes for health and well-being in midlife
Child abuse	Increased vulnerability to drug abuse, sexual risk-taking, mental health problems, psychiatric disorders, offending and anti-social behaviour
Insecure parental attachments and unresponsive parenting	Poorer mental health and emotional well-being, as well as experiencing unsuccessful relationships in adulthood
Poverty	This has been linked to increased risks of cardiovascular disease, obesity and Type 2 diabetes in adulthood, as well as to lower educational attainment, employment and socioeconomic status

Risks in adolescence

Chronic illnesses	Legacies of fertility, emotional and developmental problems, serious medical conditions, ongoing anxiety, reduced employment prospects, secondary cancer or treatment-related cancer, higher risk of mortality than the rest of the population
Poor mental health	Major depression, suicidal behaviour, alcoholism, anti-social personality disorders, drug misuse, as well as decreased employment opportunities, lower income, lower owner-occupation rates and increased probability of criminal activity
Anorexia nervosa and bulimia nervosa	Heart and gastrointestinal diseases, infertility, nerve damage and osteoporosis
Poor nutrition	Low levels of vegetable and fruit consumption in adolescence can increase risks of cancer and coronary heart disease
Overweight and obesity	Risk of developing sleep apnoea, high blood pressure (a major cause of strokes), high cholesterol level, hearing loss and mental illness. In addition, obesity in adolescence has been linked to many chronic diseases in adulthood that can potentially shorten the lifespan. These include diabetes, heart disease, liver disease and cancers
Inconsistent use of contraception and high number of sexual partners	Chronic illnesses, life-threatening infections and cancers due to sexually transmitted diseases contracted as a result of this sort of risk-taking behaviour in adolescence. When such risk taking resulted in the abortion of an unplanned pregnancy in adolescence, there can be an increased risk of breast cancer, pelvic inflammatory disease, depression and viral hepatitis during adulthood

Risks in adolescence	Outcomes for health and well-being in midlife
Smoking	Smoking-related illnesses in later life. Whilst the main smoking-related illness is lung cancer, it does cause other cancers such as cancer of the upper aero-digestive tract (oral cavity, nasal cavity, nasal sinuses, pharynx, larynx and oesophagus), pancreas, stomach, liver, bladder, kidney, cervix, bowel, ovary and myeloid leukaemia. Other illnesses that are recognised as being related to smoking are respiratory, vascular and chronic obstructive pulmonary diseases (COPD)
Binge drinking	Increased risk of psychological problems, cognitive impairments, ischaemic heart disease, liver disease, and the effects of irreversible brain damage and alcohol-related disorders and/or alcoholism
Regular drug use	Serious and/or persistent offending and a drug use career
Poverty and deprivation	Poorer health and well-being in general, increased risks of cardiovascular disease, obesity and Type 2 diabetes in adulthood, as well as lower educational attainment, employment and socioeconomic status

Risks in young adulthood	
Smoking	Neurological damage, a range of psychiatric disorders (for example, schizophrenia and substance abuse disorder), respiratory disease, vascular disease and chronic obstructive pulmonary disease (COPD), lung cancer and many other types of cancers such as cancer of the upper aero-digestive tract (oral cavity, nasal cavity, nasal sinuses, pharynx, larynx and oesophagus), pancreas, stomach, liver, bladder, kidney, cervix, bowel, ovary and myeloid leukaemia
Excessive alcohol consumption	Higher rates of alcohol dependence and abuse, heart disease, stroke, cancers, liver cirrhosis, amnesia, peripheral neuropathy, gastrointestinal problems, decreased bone density and blood cell production, relationship breakdown, unemployment and mortality
Recreational drug use	Psychiatric disorders, lower income, welfare dependence, unemployment, lower life satisfaction, increased risk of a drug use career, serious and/or persistent offending, relationship breakdown, unemployment, drug-related and violent death
Overweight and obesity	High blood pressure (a major cause of strokes), high cholesterol levels, hearing loss, mental illness, chronic diseases (such as heart disease and diabetes) and some cancers that can potentially shorten the lifespan

(Continued)

Table 6.1   *(Continued)*

Risks in young adulthood	Outcomes for health and well-being in midlife
Non-relationship sexual partnering	Legacies of sexually transmitted infections and unplanned pregnancies
Prolonged marital/relationship conflict	Poorer mental and physical health, including depression, psychiatric disorders, mood, anxiety and substance abuse disorders. Cardiovascular disease and mortality as a result of early onset of hypertension in young adulthood
Dissolution of intimate relationships	Physical and mental health problems, overall lower level of well-being associated with formation of new intimate relationships
Gestational diabetes in pregnancy	Development of Type 2 diabetes
Pre-eclampsia in pregnancy	Effects of a stroke, impaired kidney and liver function, blood-clotting problems, higher risk of coronary heart disease and mortality
Puerperal psychoses	Recurrent puerperal episodes that may not necessarily be related to childbearing
Early transition to parenthood	Increased risks of breast cancer, truncated educational and work opportunities, increased depression and marital instability and poorer self-rated health
Later transition to parenthood (after the age of 30)	Increased risks of breast cancer, poorer self-rated health in midlife and higher levels of depression in older life
Childlessness	Childless women have higher breast cancer rates throughout adulthood
Untreated work-related sleeping problems	High blood pressure, heart attack, stroke, Type 2 diabetes, obesity and psychiatric problems
Mental health problems	Relationship breakdown, reduced workforce participation, lower income and lower economic living standards
Undetected and untreated mental health problems	More severe and persistent symptoms of primary disorders and the development of secondary disorders and hence the accumulation of mental health problems. The outcomes are the same as for 'mental health problems', above
Long-term illnesses	The legacies of unresolved emotional problems, reduced employment. Those who had cancer in young adulthood are vulnerable to ongoing anxiety, secondary cancer or treatment-related cancer and the effects of possible infertility on their well-being
Living in a socially disadvantaged neighbourhood and experiencing poverty	Poorer physical and mental health. Examples include higher rates of cardiovascular disease, obesity, Type 2 diabetes and stress

Risks to Health and Well-Being During Midlife

Risk-taking behaviours in midlife life are generally much lower than in young adulthood; around a third of smokers quit their habit during this life stage. Other lifestyle changes that occur in midlife are more moderate alcohol consumption, lower levels of unhealthy food consumption and the cessation of illegal substance use (Berger, 2011). Whilst lifestyle factors will be explored in this section, as we will see, in addition to the impact of risks to health and well-being from previous stages (as shown in Table 6.1) new risks to health and well-being arise that are specific to this life stage.

The grid set out below uses the same format as that in Table 6.1. As you read through the rest of this section, try to identify any risks that are likely to affect health and well-being in old age. Make a note of them on the grid and then compare them with those in Table 7.1 in Chapter 7. This activity is designed to help you continue to develop your ability to interpret the findings about health and well-being at a particular life stage from a life course perspective.

ACTIVITY 6.1

Risks in midlife	Outcomes for health and well-being in old age

Lifestyle

Although risk-taking behaviour is lower in midlife, lifestyles can still threaten longer-term health. Those who smoke, have low levels of physical activity and do not drink in moderation, eat healthily and maintain a normal weight are at increased risk of a wide range of diseases and shortened lifespan (Appel, 2005; Nusselder et al., 2009; Ruidavets et al., 2010).

Let us look in more detail at the effects of some of these lifestyle factors in midlife. Alcohol use plateaus in middle age, and from late middle age onwards the course of alcohol consumption and drinking problems is one of net decline.

Moderate drinking in midlife has several health benefits; those who drink moderately experience less stress and depression as well as lower mortality than either abstainers or heavy drinkers. However, recent studies have shown that there is an increase in the number in this age group who drink over the 'recommended' weekly amounts of alcohol, and in alcohol-related deaths (Littlefield and Sher, 2010; Brennan et al., 2011; Emslie et al., 2011). Alcohol dependence and harmful use of alcohol in midlife threatens health during the rest of the life course; research shows that it results in increased risk of heart disease, stroke, cancers, and liver cirrhosis, amnesia, cognitive deficits, sleep problems, peripheral neuropathy, gastrointestinal problems and decreased bone density and blood-cell production (Schuckit, 2009).

Smoking in itself in midlife increases the risk of a range of diseases (for example, cancers, heart diseases and chronic obstructive pulmonary disease (COPD)) but smoking *and* drinking increase mortality rates significantly (Geijer et al., 2006; Hart et al., 2010). Low levels of physical activity in midlife also increase the risk of cancer and heart disease. However, a recent study found that the effects of lower levels of physical activity in early middle age could be counteracted by engaging in higher levels in later middle age; those who increased their activity levels between the ages of 50 and 65 ended up living as long as those who were already exercising regularly by middle age (Orsini et al., 2008).

With reference to weight control, excess weight in middle age can influence the degradation of the brain, increase risk of cancer, heart diseases, vascular diseases, **dementia** and spending many years of life with a disability (Klijs et al., 2011; Xu et al., 2011). Those entering middle age who are overweight or obese are already at risk of chronic diseases such as heart disease, cancer, diabetes, strokes, high blood pressure and mental illness. They may also be experiencing poorer social and economic conditions (Finch and Searle, 2005; Kuh et al., 2005; *Foresight Report*, 2007). Even if individuals have previously maintained a healthy weight, midlife is a time of life when people are likely to gain weight. This is because between the ages of 20 and 50 metabolism slows down by about a third. In addition, middle-aged people tend to underestimate their weight. Hence, overweight and obesity prevalence increases throughout midlife. Currently, around 70 per cent of middle-aged people are overweight or obese, which means that many at this life stage face significant threats to their health and well-being (NHS Information Centre for Health and Social Care, 2010; Rayner et al., 2010).

Relationships and Partnerships

Research about relationships and partnerships in midlife is very limited. Furthermore, it is disproportionately focused on heterosexual, White, middle-class couples and therefore does not address diversity (Sassler, 2010; Umberson et al., 2010). Nonetheless, some interesting information has emerged. For instance, higher divorce and relationship dissolution rates now mean that a substantial proportion of middle-aged adults spend more time outside of a relationship.

More people cohabit in midlife, too. As we saw in Chapter 5, those who are not married generally have poorer mental and physical health than those who are married (Fincham and Beach, 2010). With reference to midlife specifically, in comparison to married people, those who are single at this life stage have been found to be at greater risk of Human Immunodeficiency Virus (HIV), less happy than those who are married and more likely to develop dementia between the ages of 65 and 79 (Hunt, 2005; McCormick et al., 2009; Health Protection Agency, 2011). Although those who cohabit have less depression than single people in this age group, they do experience more depression than married people. Those who experience dissolution of their marital and non-marital relationships in midlife have more symptoms of depression and anxiety and higher rates of substance abuse. In addition to such mental health problems, their physical health is more likely to be threatened both during middle adulthood and in later life, for instance they are more at risk of cardiovascular disease. Therefore, their overall mortality rates are also higher (Zhang and Hayward, 2006; Amato, 2010; Bracke et al., 2010; Heffner at al., 2011).

As a consequence of marital and non-marital relationship dissolution, many individuals in midlife will also be in new intimate relationships that often involve the formation of remarried families and stepfamilies. We saw in the last chapter how these relationships can be challenging and stressful because they are built on existing foundations of partnership, parenthood and extended kin relationship. This is particularly so when they involve parenting children of different biological relatedness. As a result, those who remarry tend to have lower levels of well-being at any stage in life and the length of second and subsequent marriages is shorter when compared with first marriages (Green, 2010; Sassler, 2010; Sweeney, 2010; Umberson et al., 2010).

Another development in relationships and partnerships in midlife is the increasing number of children born to women over 40 (referred to above); three times as many children were born to women over 40 in 2010 than in 1990 (Office for National Statistics, 2009a, 2011a). Whilst there are many rewards for older parents, they have to cope with the stresses and strains of caring for young children (see Chapter 5) with considerably less energy than younger parents. Indeed, transition into parenthood in midlife is associated with more depressive symptoms (Carlson, 2011). Moreover, advanced maternal and parental age is associated with a higher risk of a child being born with Down syndrome, autism and decreased intellectual capacity. Parenting a child with a disorder can lead to reduced employment opportunities, physical and emotional stress, depressive symptoms, feelings of isolation and high levels of anxiety. These concurrent outcomes can also impact on later physical and mental health (McConkey et al., 2008; Eisenhower et al., 2009; Benzies et al., 2011; Venter, 2011).

However, for a significant proportion of people in midlife, parenthood involves parenting teenage and adult children. The turbulence of adolescence inevitably means a certain amount of conflict in most families. Where this is frequent and protracted, parents are likely to experience stress and depressive symptoms not only during their child's adolescence but in later life, too. These symptoms are more severe when violence occurs during parent–adolescent conflict (Mitchell and Hauser-Cram, 2008; Holt, 2011; Milkie et al., 2011). There is now a body of evidence to support the view that 'parenthood is a role that never ends' and that even when parenthood and parenting involve adult children it shapes life experiences and has 'significant effects on psychological and physical well-being over the life course', and 'emotionally close and supportive ties with adult children enhance parents' well-being, whereas strained and conflicted relationships with children undermine well-being' (Umberson et al., 2010: 618–19).

Whilst worse than expected relationships with adult children are associated with lower well-being (Umberson et al., 2010), a parent's marital status has been found to influence the nature of the relationship with his or her adult children and hence the extent that these relationships can potentially enhance or undermine parental well-being. Divorced and widowed mothers seem to benefit most from closer and more supportive relationships with adult children. In contrast, divorced fathers have more distant and strained relationships with adult children that can lead to decreased well-being. Interestingly, childlessness in midlife is not associated with worse psychological outcomes than parenthood at this life stage. Furthermore, there is some evidence that middle-aged people who do not have children have less depression and higher levels of social activity than parents at the same life stage (Umberson et al., 2010).

A very significant event in parenting teenage and adult children is when they leave the parental home. The set of reactions that occur at this time are referred to as the 'empty nest syndrome'. Some parents find it difficult and react negatively to their perceived state of disequilibrium; such reactions include overwhelming grief, sadness, **dysporia**, depression and loss of identity. These parents tend to find the personal and family adjustments required very challenging and an 'empty nest' can therefore add to the 'crisis' of this time in the life course. However, other parents successfully adjust by creating their own meanings, renewing marital relationships, forging new identities and engaging in new activities. Influences on these reactions include personality, age cohort, societal emphasis on the maternal role, workforce participation and the development of alternative roles (Crowley et al., 2003; Hunt, 2005; Asthana, 2010; Berger, 2011).

ACTIVITY 6.2

Preeti and Lauri

The following case study presents a very positive view of life for parents once their children have left 'the nest'. As you read, think about the sorts of factors that would influence the extent to which an 'empty nest' can be as rewarding as described in the article:

Preeti and Lauri are both in their early fifties. When the last of their three children, Asha, recently left home to work abroad, they had worried that they would suffer from 'empty-nest syndrome'. Another couple with whom they had been friends for a number of years found that the departure of their children meant that the one thing that they had in common had gone and their relationship had sadly ended. However, six months after Asha's departure, Preeti and Lauri were physically and mentally fitter than they had been for years. As they were no longer having to support any of their children financially and had let out one of the children's rooms, they were nearly £600 a month better off. They also had far more free time because there was less ironing, cooking and tidying up to do. With both more money and time, they were socialising with friends at least twice a week and had already taken three foreign holidays and had another one planned for the following month. Preeti was pursuing her interests in cookery and alternative medicine at an evening class. Lauri had taken up his artwork again after a break of many years and had joined a local art group. Being able to spend more quality time together had also improved their relationship.

Some people become grandparents in midlife. Whilst most find this an affirming and emotionally fulfilling experience which helps them to 'feel young again', there is a sense of ambiguity around grandparenthood because of the lack of clearly defined norms about this role. This is especially the case for those grandparents who are not closely involved in their grandchildren's lives. This ambiguity is compounded by stepgrandparenting; rates of remarriage and the growth of reconstituted families mean that this is an increasing phenomenon (Hunt, 2005; Berger, 2011). Grandparents who parent their grandchildren, for whatever reason, tend to have worse physical health than those who do not, as well as more social and financial problems (Umberson et al., 2010).

How are you doing with your grid? Here are some suggestions about points that you could have included so far for you to check out.

ACTIVITY 6.3

Risks in midlife	Outcomes for health and well-being in old age
Alcohol dependence and harmful use of alcohol	Shortened lifespan in general because of increased risk of heart disease, stroke, cancers, and liver cirrhosis, amnesia, cognitive deficits, sleep problems, peripheral neuropathy, gastrointestinal problems, decreased bone density and blood cell production
Smoking	Increases the risk of cancer, heart diseases and chronic obstructive pulmonary disease (COPD)
Smoking and drinking alcohol	Increase mortality rates significantly
Low levels of physical activity	Increases risk of cancer and heart diseases

(Continued)

(Continued)

Risks in midlife	Outcomes for health and well-being in old age
Excess weight in middle age	Degradation of the brain, increased risk of cancer, diabetes, heart diseases, vascular diseases, dementia, strokes, high blood pressure, mental illness and spending many years with a disability. This may also lead to poorer social and economic conditions
Intimate relationship dissolutions and/or living alone	Greater risk of more physical and mental health problems generally, and depression and dementia specifically. Overall, mortality is also higher
Strained relationships with children	Depressive symptoms
Parenting grandchildren	Poorer physical health

Male and Female Menopause

As we saw earlier in the chapter, some critics claim that the female menopause has been increasingly medicalised. Others have argued that it is socially constructed, pointing to the evidence of cultural variations in women's experiences of the menopause and the fact that psychological symptoms of the menopause may be the result of concurrent events in women's lives in particular cultures. Indeed, not only is there a lack of consensus about the psychological symptoms but there is also some dissension about the biological symptoms; examples of the latter include the way in which hot flushes and headaches are the most common symptoms of menopause amongst Western women whereas Japanese women are most likely to report constipation and diarrhoea (Hardy and Kuh, 2002; Hunt, 2005). Nonetheless, both sets of symptoms can be very distressing. Many women also find that their moods change inexplicably from day to day. However, clinical depression is rare during the menopause, except in women who already have a history of depression. Onset of symptoms is variable; the sudden onset of the menopause caused by a hysterectomy is likely to produce more dramatic biological and psychological symptoms (Green, 2010; Berger, 2011). Timing of the menopause has implications for health in the shorter and the longer term. Early menopause is associated with an increased risk of osteoporosis and cardiovascular disease whilst later menopause has been linked to an increased risk of breast cancer. Furthermore, the reduction in hormone levels that occurs results in increased fat deposits in the arteries and loss of bone calcium. Both of these can have more serious consequences in that increased fat deposits in the arteries can set the stage for coronary heart disease, and loss of bone calcium can eventually lead to osteoporosis (Hardy and Kuh, 2002; Rich-Edwards, 2002).

When discussing the male menopause above we saw how the existence of this is contentious, not least within the medical profession. Those who argue for its existence use the terms 'andropause' and 'manopause' and point to evidence of progressive changes in male hormone levels in midlife and how these can lead to irritability, depression, fatigue and loss of libido. Others argue that 'much still remains unproven' (Hunt, 2005: 176) and attribute its emergence to the 'public's belief that medicine could cure any condition' from the 1950s onwards (Green, 2010: 153).

Employment

Job loss in midlife (particularly 55 plus) is higher than in younger age groups and re-employment chances are usually poor. Both worry about job loss and job loss itself increase depression levels. When unemployment does occur in midlife it often leads to poorer diet and low life satisfaction. It can also lead to depressive symptoms in spouses (Economic and Social Research Council, 2011; Mandal et al., 2011; Dave and Kelly, 2012). Although burnout decreases with age during midlife, work-related and life situational factors mean that burnout in this age group has been found to be higher for women than for men (Norlund et al., 2010). Despite the fact that many middle-aged people yearn for retirement, there is considerable debate about the influence of the timing of retirement on health. Studies have shown that although there is an association between early retirement and reduced subsequent risk of depressive symptoms and fatigue, there is some evidence that that those who retire early (for example, at 55) have higher mortality rates than those who retire at 65. They also have higher suicide rates. Whilst the increased suicide risk is independent of categorised psychiatric diagnosis, the higher mortality rates could be because some of those who retire early do so on health grounds (Burdorf, 2010; Rice et al., 2011; Schneider et al., 2011).

Caring

Midlife is a time when people are most likely to have to care for their elderly parents. A growing number of middle-aged people combine providing this informal care with dealing with the demands of adult children and employment (Green, 2010; Eldh and Carlsson, 2011). Whilst being a carer is rewarding in many ways, it can place considerable demands on carers that are compounded when there are pressures from other sources, such as unaccommodating employers. The gendered nature of caring suggests that it is 'midlife women who may be experiencing considerable time famine and stress with their multiple roles and burdens' (Green, 2010: 169). Studies over a number of years have shown that caring affects physical and psychological health. For instance, carers experience a wide range of problems such as depression, anxiety, emotional distress, stress, feeling tired, hernias, heart problems, arthritis, asthma, giddiness, backaches and headaches. Caring may also impact negatively on personal and sexual relationships, employment opportunities, financial and social circumstances, self-confidence, self-esteem and identity (Yeandle et al., 2007; Larkin, 2011b).

As explained at the very beginning of this chapter, midlife is the stage in our lives when mental distress decreases. However, there is evidence that the risk of mental health problems is increasing for some middle-aged people more than for others. Read through the following extract from a recent newspaper article. As you read, think about the following questions:

1   According to the findings in the article, which group of middle-aged people is experiencing an increase in mental health problems?
2   What factors are identified as contributing towards this increase?
3   Which of these factors were addressed in the discussions of the possible risks to health and well-being during midlife in this section of the chapter?

There are some suggestions about the answers to help you at the end of the chapter.

One in four women aged between 45 and 64 now experience some form of mental disorder – an increase of 20 per cent in the last 15 years. This decline in mental health is greater than in any other age or gender group, according to the research. The mental health charity Mind said that women in their forties and fifties were becoming increasingly affected by trying to manage the responsibilities of family, home and work. The NHS Information Centre report (2009) titled the *Adult Psychiatric Morbidity in England, 2007*, was carried out by the National Centre for Social Research and the University of Leicester and questioned 7461 adults. It followed on from two similar NHS studies carried out in England in 1993 and 2000. The report concluded that the number of 45- to 64-year-old women with a common mental disorder rose from 20.5 per cent in 1993 to 25.2 per cent in 2007. The survey also found that the number of women aged between 16 and 74 who reported having suicidal thoughts in the previous year rose from 4.2 per cent in 2000 to 5.5 per cent in 2007. Peter Byrne, Director of Public Education at the Royal College of Psychiatrists, said that the role of women had changed significantly in the last 15 years. 'This particular age group was probably reared by their stay-at-home mothers and they are almost certainly now working mothers, who face the financial pressure of being part of a two-income family' and yet it is still accepted 'that when elderly parents fall ill, the responsibility always falls on the daughter'. Paul Farmer, Chief Executive of Mind, said that the stigma still surrounding mental health may be preventing women from getting help. 'It is worrying that we have seen such a large increase in the number of middle-aged women experiencing mental health problems such as depression and anxiety,' he said. 'Today's women in their 40s and 50s face numerous responsibilities such as caring for elderly relatives, looking after young children or teenagers and managing a full-time career. Juggling all of these roles can be a heavy burden to bear and can send stress levels soaring. Women may be finding it difficult to take time out for themselves to take care of their own mental well-being but it's vital that they take their mental health just as seriously as they would their physical health' (Gammell, 2009).

Finished your grid? Now look at the risks that are likely to affect health and well-being in young adulthood in Table 6.1 with those that you have identified in relation to midlife your grid. Are there any differences? If so, why do you think that these differences exist?

ACTIVITY 6.5

Negative *and* Positive Influences on the Risks to Health and Well-Being in Midlife

As explained in previous chapters, health and well-being at each life stage not only depend on the cumulative effects of risks from previous life stages and risks to health and well-being at that life stage itself but also on a variety of interacting factors that influence the impact of these risks. An example of these factors that has emerged from the discussions about risks to health and well-being in middle age is the way in which gender shapes the experience of caring in midlife. Another example is the way in which social and demographic changes, such as increases in marital and non-marital relationship dissolutions and the numbers of reconstituted families, can potentially undermine well-being. In addition to understanding these influences on the risks to health and well-being in midlife, the life course approach argues that it is very important to take into consideration both negative *and* positive influences as the latter can have the 'protective effects' (Bryant et al., 2003: 363) referred to earlier in the chapter. With reference to positive influences, studies on the risks to health and well-being in midlife show that a good level of income in young and middle adulthood can compensate for some of the longer-term effects on health and well-being of poverty and disadvantage in childhood (Tucker-Seeley et al., 2011). Likewise, personality type and culture can have positive effects on health and well-being at this life stage; those who are self-transcendent, creative and optimistic cope better with midlife. Women who live in cultures in which the menopause is viewed positively report 'fewer physical and mental symptoms' (Green, 2010: 152) (Hardy and Kuh, 2002; Green, 2010). Other more positive influences are certain cultural changes; the enhanced well-being of those without children has been associated with shifts in cultural attitudes that have shaped the 'meaning, experience and consequences of childlessness' (Umberson et al., 2010: 3). As a result of these changes, parenthood is increasingly viewed as a matter of choice and voluntary childlessness has become much more common. Hence, those who choose not to have children are less likely to be subjected to the negative cultural and societal attitudes towards childlessness that have existed. However, it is important to note that involuntary childlessness can be the cause of much distress throughout the life course. Therefore, heterogeneity among the childless needs to be taken into consideration when exploring cultural influences on the experience of childlessness (Umberson et al., 2010).

The variables that have a more negative influence on the risks to health and well-being in midlife are similar to those identified in other chapters. These are explored in the rest of this section. As you will see, the outcomes of these variables are shaped by the particular characteristics of this life stage.

Gender

The article in Activity 6.4 points out that women in midlife are often very pressurised as they have many roles to 'juggle', such as managing a home and a fulltime career, caring for elderly parents and looking after young children and/or teenagers. Indeed, there is a growing body of evidence that shows that women are more likely to experience time famine, exhaustion and burnout levels than men at this life stage (Green, 2010; Norlund et al., 2010; Lindeberg et al., 2011). Furthermore, many recent studies have shown that being female increases a number of the risks to health and well-being in midlife that were discussed in the previous section. With reference to the increase in those in this age group who drink over the 'recommended' weekly amounts of alcohol, this has been most notable amongst women (Emslie et al., 2011). However, being a male also has its disadvantages in middle age; although the survey referred to in Activity 6.4 found that the number of women aged between 16 and 74 who reported having suicidal thoughts in the previous year had risen, research has shown that it is men who are more likely to have suicidal thoughts at this life stage than women (Hunt et al., 2006). Men have also been found to have fewer longstanding friendships (Green, 2010).

Poverty and Social Disadvantage

The association between poverty and social disadvantage in midlife and poorer health and well-being in general has been established for some time (Kuh and Wadsworth, 1993; Rayner et al., 2010; Platt, 2011). Specific conditions highlighted in the literature are higher blood pressure, a greater risk of dementia and higher rates of obesity and coronary heart disease (Beauchamp et al., 2011; Loucks et al., 2011). Poverty and social disadvantage also increase the risk of other threats to health and well-being. Examples are the way in which poverty increases marital and familial conflict and, in turn, the risk of divorce (Amato, 2010; Fincham and Beach, 2010; Marmot Review Team, 2011). Although upward social mobility is protective to health, if those who are advantaged in middle age had previously been socially and economically disadvantaged, they do 'not attain the same levels of health as those who were advantaged over the whole life course' (Davey Smith and Lynch, 2005: 97). Similarly, those whose income in midlife is much lower than the average for someone with the same level of education or in the same occupation are more prone to cardiovascular disease in midlife (Braig et al., 2011). This mismatch between status indicators is known as **status inconsistency**.

Some of the aforementioned conditions (such as hypertension, obesity and coronary heart disease) can be attributed to the negative influence that poverty and social disadvantage have on midlife lifestyle choices. The most notable of these are the adoption of harmful patterns of alcohol consumption, higher smoking rates, lower rates of physical activity and weight control (Batty et al., 2008; Rayner et al., 2010; Boone-Heinonen et al., 2011; Giskes et al., 2011). However, there is recent evidence that this is partly due to the fact that adherence to lifestyle behaviour is long term and there is a strong relationship between unhealthy lifestyles and poorer socioeconomic circumstances. Hence, those living in adverse social circumstances in middle age who have also experienced poverty and disadvantage at earlier life stages are more likely to be 'locked into' an unhealthy lifestyle than those who have not (Rees Jones et al., 2011).

Discussion Point

What are the advantages and disadvantages of the life course approach to health and well-being in middle adulthood? What other approaches could be useful?

Prevention, Prevention, Prevention …

The general lack of distinction between young and middle adulthood in the literature limits the extent of any analysis of policy initiatives aimed at improving health and well-being in midlife specifically. Nonetheless, it is clear that the main themes in national and international initiatives that address the needs of those in this life stage are health screening, health prevention and early interventions to reduce the incidence of chronic diseases and mental illnesses. With reference to chronic diseases, as explained earlier in the chapter (see p. 108), there has been a particular emphasis on cancer screening, and monitoring blood pressure, weight and cholesterol. The focus in these health prevention initiatives has been on lifestyle modification. Physical exercise, smoking, alcohol consumption, diet and weight loss have received particular attention (National Institute for Health and Clinical Excellence, 2006, 2007b; Busse et al., 2011; Gray et al., 2011). As a consequence, some innovative programmes have been introduced. Amongst these are exercise referral schemes and the use of software programmes for those with unhealthy drinking habits (Hester et al., 2005; National Institute for Health and Clinical Excellence, 2006; Gray et al., 2011). Other initiatives are aimed at reducing the risk of certain chronic diseases, such as cardiovascular diseases (Brekke and Straand, 2011). There have also been many attempts to evaluate these schemes. Few have proved to produce the intended outcomes, and research to identify ways in which they can result in better health and well-being as well as be cost effective is ongoing (Hillsdon et al., 2005; Anokye et al., 2011). An analysis of the wider problem of motivating people to alter their lifestyles is presented in the quotation below:

> A genetic predisposition to disease is difficult to alter. Social circumstances can also be difficult to change, at least in the short to medium term. By comparison, people's behaviour – as individuals and collectively – may be easier to change. However, many attempts to do this have been unsuccessful, or only partially successful. Often, this has been because they fail to take account of the theories and principles of successful planning, delivery and evaluation. At present, there is no strategic approach to behaviour change across government, the NHS or other sectors, and many different models, methods and theories are being used in an uncoordinated way. (National Institute for Health and Clinical Excellence, 2007b: 6)

Hence, there is a need for a revised approach to lifestyle change in policies that target chronic illness in midlife. A range of interventions in the area of mental health promotion, prevention and early intervention has also been developed that includes improvements in the mental health of those in midlife. However, it has been argued that improving mental health 'will depend less on specific interventions, valuable as these may be' (Friedli, 2009: iv) and more on the adoption of a new approach. This is illustrated in the following extract from a recent Department of Health publication about mental health:

> The Government has a new approach. ... this new approach to government means a different approach to direction setting – developing strategies to achieve outcomes. Outcomes strategies reject the top-down approach of the past. Instead, they focus on how people can best be empowered to lead the lives they want to lead and to keep themselves and their families healthy, to learn and be able to work in safe and resilient communities, and on how practitioners on the front line can best be supported to deliver what matters to service users within an ethos that maintains dignity and respect. (Department of Health, 2011c: 10)

Clearly, revisiting existing approaches and identifying and implementing alternative evidence-based approaches is a priority if the risks to health and well-being during midlife are to be reduced.

Conclusions

In this chapter we have seen how risks from previous life stages can accumulate and impact on health and well-being in midlife. The impact of these accumulated risks and threats to health and well-being at this life stage is unpredictable as it depends on many complicated interactions between a number of variables. In the 'Conclusions' to each of the chapters in this book that have addressed a specific life stage (namely, Chapters 2, 3, 4 and 5), there has been a reflection on the extent to which the material discussed supports Graham's view that pregnancy, childhood and adolescence are 'an unparalleled time during which external influences, both good and bad, can influence an individual's health and well-being across their whole life' (Graham, 2009: 26). Once again, empirical verification of this claim in relation to midlife is not possible. Nonetheless, the evidence presented has shown that not only do 'pregnancy, childhood and adolescence' have a considerable influence on health and well-being in midlife but what happens in middle adulthood is also of consequence. This indicates that significant risks to health and well-being continue to accumulate post-adolescence. The final part of our assessment of Graham's argument necessitates an exploration of health and well-being in old age. This is the topic of the next chapter.

Summary

- Whilst our general health declines throughout midlife, this is the stage in our lives when levels of mental distress decrease
- Weight gain, obesity and increasing susceptibility to osteoporosis are all health issues in midlife. Those over 50 are at the highest risk of cancer. The most common cancers are breast cancers in women and prostate, lung and colorectal cancers in men
- Evidence from other chapters about the cumulative nature of risks to health and well-being throughout the life course clearly shows that there are more threats to our health and well-being in midlife from previous life stages than in any of the life stages discussed so far in this book. Nonetheless, the extent to which these risks become reality depends on a range of interacting variables that influence them both positively and negatively
- Risks to health and well-being during midlife include lifestyle factors (such as smoking, low levels of physical activity, immoderate drinking and failure to maintain a normal weight), relationship status, transition into parenthood in midlife, parenting children of different biological relatedness, teenage children, adult children and grandchildren, male and female menopause, employment and being an unpaid carer
- Examples of positive influences on these risks to health and well-being during midlife are a good level of income in young and middle adulthood, personality type and culture. Amongst the more negative influences are gender, poverty and social disadvantage
- Initiatives aimed at improving health and well-being in midlife have focused on health screening and health prevention. Less than ideal outcomes in relation to lifestyle modification have led to an ongoing search for effective solutions

Further Study

Although there is a relative dearth of literature about health and well-being in midlife, several of the *Lifespan* books have chapters dedicated to each life stage. An example is K. Berger, *The Developing Person through the Lifespan*, 8th edn (New York: Worth Publishers, 2011). Chapter 8 in S. Hunt, *The Life Course: A Sociological Introduction* (Basingstoke: Palgrave Macmillan, 2005), provides a sociological perspective on the way in which midlife has been problematised. If you are particularly interested in women's health, many of the chapters in D. Kuh and R. Hardy (eds), *A Life Course Approach to Women's Health* (Oxford: Oxford University Press, 2002), make significant contributions to our understanding of women's health and well-being in midlife.

Activity Comments

Ideas to help you with this activity are in italics after each of the questions below:

1   According to the findings in the article, which group of middle-aged people is experiencing an increase in mental health problems? – *Women aged between 45 and 64, although there is also evidence of an increase in the number of women aged between 16 and 74 who reported having suicidal thoughts*
2   What factors are identified as contributing towards this increase in the extract? – *Managing a home and fulltime career, caring for elderly parents, looking after young children or teenagers*
3   Which of these factors were addressed in the discussions of the possible risks to health and well-being during midlife in this section of the chapter? – *All of them*

7

Health and Well-Being in Old Age

Introduction

The social category of 'old age' is a socially constructed and relative concept. It is also extremely broad and in some contexts it is not even referred to as such – the terms 'late adulthood', the 'last decades of life' or 'The Third Age' being deemed preferable alternatives. In addition, many people designated as elderly do not self-identify as 'old'. However, for statistical and policy purposes, people over 65 are classified as being 'older people'. Those who are over 85 are often referred to as 'old old' (Degnen, 2007). The data about health and well-being across the life course presented in Chapter 1 clearly shows that we experience our worst health in old age – this is a time in life when the number of those reporting that their health is 'not good' is at its highest. The incidence of acute, chronic and mental illnesses also peaks in old age with the sharpest increases in those over 75. Indeed, older people account for a high proportion of hospitalisations, including multiple hospital admissions (Sona et al., 2012). Other distinctive features of this life stage include the way in which its endpoint is not defined chronologically and it can be one of the longest life stages. The former is obviously attributable to the fact that the length of individual lifespans after the age of 65 varies considerably. Increasing longevity contributes to the variability of the latter; average life expectancy has increased dramatically over the past 100 years. In 1901, this was 45 for males and 49 for females. By 2002, it was 76 and 81 for males and females, respectively, and these figures are projected to rise to 93 and 97, respectively, by 2056 (Office for National Statistics, 2008). Therefore, health and well-being in old age is more likely to be alterable at this life stage than at any other time in the life course because of its sheer length. Add to this the natural heterogeneity amongst older people and you will begin to appreciate the complexity of health and well-being during old age.

This chapter not only aims to capture this complexity but also to provide further insights into health and well-being in old age by using the life course approach. Following an outline of the main changes in health and well-being that occur during old age, the chapter looks at the role of the cumulative risks and experiences from conception through to infancy, childhood, adolescence, young adulthood and middle adulthood. It then addresses risks to the health and well-being of older people. As this is the last stage in the life course, it is obviously impossible to interpret these from a life course perspective in terms of the extent to which these impact on health and well-being in future life stages. Therefore, in contrast to other chapters in this book, the focus will be on the evidence that these risks increase and accumulate, alone and in combination with risk factors in preceding life stages, throughout this life stage. Factors that influence the outcomes of these risks are discussed in the penultimate section of the chapter. The last section assesses policy initiatives that have attempted to reduce the risks and make old age a more positive experience. As in the other chapters in this book, there will be a reflection on the evidence presented in relation to the argument that 'pregnancy, childhood and adolescence' have an 'unparalleled' (Graham, 2009: 26) influence on our health and well-being across our whole life.

Health and Well-Being in Old Age

Old age is characterised by irreversible physical and cognitive changes. Physical changes include hair pigment turning grey and ultimately white, body hair thinning, skin becoming drier, thinner, less elastic and with the appearance of age spots, blood vessels becoming more visible, decreased muscle flexibility and energy, delayed reaction time and reduced mobility. The distribution of our fat changes, too – it tends to relocate itself in the torso and lower face. Our **vital organs** become less effective and slower. There is also a dulling of the senses; these include our sense of touch (especially at the extremities), taste and smell as well as the more critical senses of sight and hearing. Amongst the cognitive changes that take place are deteriorating short-term memory and speed of information processing (World Health Organization, 2002; Beckett, 2009; Green, 2010).

Poor health and well-being often accompany these changes. Even though life expectancy has increased, not all of the years gained are lived in good health. Indeed, 'healthy life expectancy, that is expected years of life in "good" or "fairly good" health, is lower than overall life expectancy' (Allen, 2008: 9). For example, research shows that although a baby boy born in 2004 had a life expectancy of 76.6, he can only expect to live in good health for 67.9 years and to be free of any form of disability for 62.3 years. Consequently, he can expect 8.7 years in poor health and 14.3 years with a disability of some sort. Similarly, a baby girl born in 2004 had a life expectancy of 81 but she is only likely to enjoy good health for 70.3 years and to be disability-free up until she is 63.9. This is because it is estimated that the last 10.7 years of her life will be spent in poor health and she will have 17.1 years with a disability. This is illustrated in Table 7.1.

Table 7.1   Life expectancy, healthy life expectancy and disability-free life expectancy in the United Kingdom, by sex, 2004

	Males		**Females**	
	At birth	**At age 65**	**At birth**	**At age 65**
Life expectancy	76.6	16.6	81	19.4
Healthy life expectancy	67.9	12.5	70.3	14.5
Years spent in poor health	8.7	4.1	10.7	4.9
Disability-free life expectancy	62.3	9.9	63.9	10.7
Years spent with disability	14.3	6.7	17.1	8.7

Source: Allen (2008: 9).

Indeed, as explained in the Introduction, poor health and well-being are more common in old age than in any other life stage. For instance, with reference to the more critical senses mentioned above, whilst most vision problems can be corrected by wearing glasses, about 10 per cent of people over 65 develop serious vision problems, such as **cataracts, glaucoma** and **age-related macular degeneration**. About 40 per cent are affected by age-related hearing loss that is known medically as **presbycusis**. Despite the fact that diseases in general advance at slower rates than in younger years, the incidence of hypertension, heart disease, strokes, diabetes, arteriosclerosis and cancer is higher in older age. Using cancer an example, over half (53 per cent) of all cancers are diagnosed in 50- to 74-year-olds. The most common cancers for males are lung, prostate and colorectal cancer. Breast cancer and lung cancer are amongst those most frequently experienced by females (NHS Information Centre for Health and Social Care, 2011). In addition, many older people suffer from mental health problems such as clinical depression, sleep disorders, anxiety, delirium, dementia, schizophrenia and alcohol and drug abuse (Lowry et al., 2007; Allen, 2008; Berger, 2011). Prevalence rates for these mental health problems could be even higher because of 'a significant degree of under-reporting of mental health problems among older people' (McCormick et al., 2009: 7). Of further concern is the rise in the number of older people with mental disorders and the predicted national and international doubling of the number of people with dementia and **Alzheimer's disease** (the most common form of dementia) over the next 20 years (Ferri et al., 2006; McCrone et al., 2008; NHS Information Centre for Health and Social Care, 2009). New health problems in old age have also emerged with developments in medical treatments for these conditions. The earlier diagnosis and more effective therapies now available that slow the progression of dementia means that older people will remain in the early stages of dementia for longer. Although independent living is possible, they do experience considerable emotional turmoil and problems with cognitive loss in these early stages (Steeman et al., 2007; Allen, 2008; McCrone et al., 2008).

In addition to being a time in our lives when poor health and well-being are more common, old age is also a time of 'deteriorating health' (Victor et al., 2009: 88). There have been some attempts to identify stages of old age in relation to the degree of ill health that is experienced. Zarrit's (1996) work is an example of one such attempt; he uses the term 'young old' for the earlier part of old age when people are independent and active and in relatively good health. This mainly occurs between 60 and 75. 'The middle old' is the transitional period between independence and dependency where individuals' physical and mental functions and health begin to deteriorate. Those whom Zarrit refers to as 'old old' are at last stage of old age and are very dependent and have numerous difficulties and high support needs. There is a considerable body of evidence to support the use of such categories in order to describe the deterioration in health and well-being that occurs in old age. For instance, the sharpest increases in mental health problems in older people occur in those over 85. Those over 80 are far more likely to suffer multimorbidity as a result of a variety of degenerative and age-related diseases such as dementia, arthritis, osteoporosis, heart conditions and cancer. As a consequence, two-thirds of people over 85 have a long-term illness or disability. Such health problems inevitably lead to them being more likely to be dependent (Larkin, 2009; Cancer Research UK, 2011; Katz et al., 2011; NHS Information Centre for Health and Social Care, 2011).

Hence, the age of older people can lead to heterogeneity in their health and well-being. Furthermore, many older people confound chronological assumptions as evidenced by the way in which a significant proportion of older people, particularly those under 74, do enjoy good health, take up new interests, do voluntary work and lead independent and healthy active lives (Larkin, 2009). Whilst some of the heterogeneity can be accounted for by genetics, according to the life course approach we need to start by examining the contribution of cumulative risks to health and well-being prior to old age (Green, 2010; Platt, 2011). This is addressed in the next section of this chapter.

Life Before Old Age

The cumulative risks from all of the life stages that precede old age identified in the reviews of research and literature in this book are summarised in Table 7.2. The sheer volume of the findings about risks to health and well-being across the life course and the speed at which they are emerging renders capturing all relevant information an impossibility. However, Table 7.2 validates the assertion from the life course perspective that health outcomes are cumulative.

As explained in previous chapters, the risks that we are exposed to at earlier life stages do not necessarily threaten our health and well-being in old age as they can be mediated by a number of interacting variables, some of which have 'protective effects'. Variables that impact on health and well-being in midlife that were discussed in Chapter 6 included gender, level of income and social disadvantage. We saw how some aspects of these variables increase the risk of certain threats to health and well-being whilst others have a counteracting effect. For instance, a good level of income in middle adulthood can compensate for some of the longer-term effects of poverty and disadvantage in childhood on health and well-being in midlife.

The main influences on the risks to our health and well-being in other life stages discussed in Chapters 2 to 6 are parental influences, poverty and social disadvantage, culture, gender, the economy and personality. Poverty and social disadvantage generally have a negative effect on health and well-being in all of the life stages. Moreover, research has shown that exposure to hazards associated with poverty and social disadvantage (such as damp housing, smoking, inadequate nutrition in childhood and adulthood, air pollution and lack of job autonomy) across the life course leads to poorer health and well-being in early retirement (Berry, 2010). Some influences have been shown to have both positive and negative elements. Let us take the example of parental influences. In relation to styles of parenting, those who experience harsh, punitive parenting are more likely to develop depression and a range of emotional, behavioural and substance abuse problems. In contrast, those with parents who are authoritative but also warm, supportive, accepting and uncritical are more likely to have higher levels of self-esteem, as well as lower levels of depression, anxiety and behaviour and substance abuse problems. Other aspects of parenting can also have such 'protective effects', as evidenced by the findings that breastfeeding can provide protection from adverse health outcomes in adulthood, for example diabetes and coronary heart disease.

Therefore, whilst important insights can be gleaned from Table 7.2, it cannot provide a full account of health and well-being in old age from a life course perspective. Furthermore, because of the emphasis in this approach on how risks accumulate throughout the *whole* life course, an analysis of old age from a life

Table 7.2   The impact of risks to health and well-being prior to old age

Pre-pregnancy influences	Outcomes for health and well-being in old age
Maternal pre-pregnancy weight below 50 kg	This can lead to low birth weight, which in turn can result in a range of adverse health outcomes in adulthood, such as cardiovascular diseases, hypertension and diabetes
Fetal exposures	
Low-quality maternal diet	Poor fetal growth and low birth weight that can result in cardiovascular diseases, hypertension, obesity and diabetes
Obesity in pregnancy	Increases risk of abnormality
Risks associated with certain foods such as uncooked meat, fish, eggs	Hydrocephalus (water on the brain), brain damage, epilepsy, deafness, blindness and growth problems
Maternal alcohol consumption	Physical and neurodevelopmental problems as a result of fetal abnormalities such as facial deformities, physical and emotional developmental problems, memory and attention deficits, as well as cognitive and behavioural problems
Prenatal stress	As this can lead to low birth weight, the risks of cardiovascular diseases, hypertension and diabetes are increased
Maternal antenatal depression	Increased vulnerability to depression and abnormalities of the neuroendocrine systems in adulthood
Uncontrolled Type 1 or Type 2 diabetes	The effects of congenital malformation
Childhood risks	
Birth trauma	The effects of irreversible brain, skeletal and organ damage that can have lifelong consequences for health and well-being. Traumatic birth experiences can also lead to childbirth-related post-traumatic stress disorder in mothers. Amongst the outcomes of such disorders is an inability to bond with the child that affects psychological health in adulthood
Maternal depression	Mental health problems as a result of the impact of maternal depression on a mother's parenting style. Maternal depression can also lead to a higher risk of infections in children up to the age of 4 years and this in turn can increase the risk of chronic diseases in adulthood, such as cardiovascular disease
Childhood illnesses	Higher rates of cancer, lung disease, cardiovascular conditions and arthritis/rheumatism have been found in adults who suffered from certain illnesses in childhood. Some conditions, such as congenital heart defects (CHD), can lead to communication and social impairment. Ill health in childhood may also have socioeconomic consequences in adulthood
Early menarche	Menarche at age 12 or less has been associated with an increased risk of breast cancer and reduced survival rate into old age

Pre-pregnancy influences	Outcomes for health and well-being in old age
Undiagnosed mental health problems	Increased vulnerability to mental health problems. Aggression in childhood that is not effectively treated is also associated with problems in adulthood such as the development of anti-social personality disorders, alcohol and drug misuse, criminality and unemployment
Passive smoking	Respiratory diseases, asthma, leukaemia, lymphoma, lung cancer and brain tumours in adulthood
Smoking	Psychological problems, respiratory diseases, vascular disease and chronic obstructive pulmonary disease (COPD), as well as many forms of cancer. The latter include lung, upper aero-digestive tract (oral cavity, nasal cavity, nasal sinuses, pharynx, larynx and oesophagus), pancreas, stomach, liver, bladder, kidney, cervix, bowel and ovarian cancer, as well as myeloid leukaemia
Diet and nutrition	An inadequate diet in childhood that contains an excess of fat and sugar intake and not enough fruit, vegetables and high-fibre products can lead to many physical and mental health problems in adulthood. Examples of these are high cholesterol, cardiovascular diseases, diabetes, high blood pressure and depression
Overweight and obesity	Risk of developing various health problems that have consequences for health-related quality of life and life expectancy in old age. These include sleep apnoea, muscularskeletal disease, diabetes, hypertension, heart disease, liver disease, pulmonary disease, some cancers, asthma and mental ill health
Being a bully	Those who are bullies in childhood are more likely to exhibit anti-social behavior in adulthood, as well as problems with maintaining stable relationships and long-term employment
Being bullied	Bullied children are at risk of being victimised in adulthood
Child abuse	Increased vulnerability to drug abuse, mental health problems, psychiatric disorders, offending and anti-social behaviour
Insecure parental attachments and unresponsive parenting	Poorer mental health and emotional well-being, and unsuccessful relationships in adulthood
Poverty	Poorer health and well-being in general, increased risks of cardiovascular disease, obesity and Type 2 diabetes in adulthood, as well as lower educational attainment, employment and socioeconomic status
Risks in adolescence	
Chronic illnesses	Legacies of reduced employment prospects, and unresolved emotional, developmental and fertility problems, serious medical conditions, ongoing anxiety, higher risks of mortality than the rest of the population
Poor mental health	Major depression, suicidal behaviour, alcoholism, anti-social personality disorders, drug misuse, as well as decreased employment opportunities, lower income, lower owner-occupation rates and increased probability of criminal activity
Anorexia nervosa and bulimia nervosa	Heart and gastrointestinal diseases, nerve damage and osteoporosis

(Continued)

Table 7.2   *(Continued)*

Risks in adolescence	Outcomes for health and well-being in old age
Poor nutrition	Low levels of vegetable and fruit consumption in adolescence can increase risks of cancer and coronary heart disease
Overweight and obesity	Risk of developing sleep apnoea, high blood pressure (a major cause of strokes), high cholesterol levels and mental illness. In addition, obesity in adolescence has been linked to many chronic diseases in adulthood that can potentially shorten the lifespan. These include diabetes, heart disease, liver disease and several different types of cancers
Inconsistent use of contraception and high number of sexual partners	Chronic illnesses, life-threatening infections and cancers due to sexually transmitted diseases contracted as a result of this sort of risk-taking behaviour in adolescence. When such risk taking resulted in the abortion of an unplanned pregnancy in adolescence, there can be an increased risk of breast cancer, pelvic inflammatory disease, depression and viral hepatitis during adulthood
Smoking	Smoking-related illnesses in later life. Whilst the main smoking-related illness is lung cancer, smoking does cause other cancers such as cancer of the upper aero-digestive tract (oral cavity, nasal cavity, nasal sinuses, pharynx, larynx and oesophagus), pancreas, stomach, liver, bladder, kidney, cervix, bowel, ovary and myeloid leukaemia. Other illnesses that are recognised as being related to smoking are respiratory, vascular and chronic obstructive pulmonary diseases
Binge drinking	Increased risk of psychological problems, cognitive impairments, ischaemic heart disease, liver disease, the effects of irreversible brain damage and alcohol-related disorders and/or alcoholism
Regular drug use	Serious and/or persistent offending and a drug-use career
Poverty and deprivation	This has been linked to poorer health and well-being in general as those who had experienced poverty during childhood and adolescence entered adulthood. More specifically, childhood poverty means increased risks of cardiovascular disease, obesity and Type 2 diabetes in adulthood, as well as lower educational attainment, employment and socioeconomic status

Risks in young adulthood	
Smoking	Neurological damage, a range of psychiatric disorders (for example, schizophrenia and substance abuse disorder), respiratory disease, vascular disease and chronic obstructive pulmonary disease, lung cancer and many other types of cancers such as cancer of the upper aero-digestive tract (oral cavity, nasal cavity, nasal sinuses, pharynx, larynx and oesophagus), pancreas, stomach, liver, bladder, kidney, cervix, bowel, ovary and myeloid leukaemia
Excessive alcohol consumption	Alcohol dependence and abuse, heart disease, stroke, cancers, and liver cirrhosis, amnesia, peripheral neuropathy, gastrointestinal problems, decreased bone density and blood cell production, loneliness (as result of relationship breakdown in previous life stages), reduced income and mortality

Risks in young adulthood	Outcomes for health and well-being in old age
Recreational drug use	Psychiatric disorders, reduced income, lower life satisfaction, drug-related death, loneliness (as result of relationship breakdown in previous life stages) and reduced income
Overweight and obesity	High blood pressure (a major cause of strokes), high cholesterol levels, hearing loss, mental illness, chronic diseases (such as heart disease and diabetes) and some cancers that can potentially shorten the lifespan
Non-relationship sexual partnering	Legacies of sexually transmitted infections and unplanned pregnancies
Intimate relationship dissolutions	Depression, anxiety, greater risk of more physical and mental health problems, lower levels of well-being because of remarriages and higher mortality rate
Gestational diabetes in pregnancy	Type 2 diabetes
Pre-eclampsia in pregnancy	Effects of a stroke, impaired kidney and liver function, blood-clotting problems, higher risk of coronary heart disease and mortality
Puerperal psychoses	Recurrent puerperal episodes unrelated to childbearing
Early transition to parenthood	Reduced income, increased risks of breast cancer and depression
Later transition to parenthood (after the age of 30)	Increased risks of breast cancer and depression
Prolonged marital/ relationship conflict	Poorer mental and physical health, including depression, psychiatric disorders, mood, anxiety and substance abuse disorders. Cardiovascular disease and mortality as result of early onset hypertension in young adulthood
Childlessness	Associated with decreased health and well-being for unmarried men and formerly married men only
Untreated work-related sleeping problems	High blood pressure, heart attack, stroke, Type 2 diabetes, obesity and psychiatric problems
Mental health problems	Loneliness (as a result of relationship breakdown in previous life stages) and reduced income
Undetected and untreated mental health problems	Accumulation of mental health problems. The outcomes of these are the same as for 'mental health problems', above

(Continued)

Table 7.2   *(Continued)*

Risks in young adulthood	Outcomes for health and well-being in old age
Long-term illnesses	The legacies of unresolved emotional problems, reduced employment. Those who had cancer in young adulthood are vulnerable to ongoing anxiety, secondary cancer or treatment-related cancer and the effects of possible infertility on their well-being
Living in a socially disadvantaged neighbourhood and experiencing poverty	Poorer physical and mental health. Examples include higher rates of cardiovascular disease, obesity, Type 2 diabetes and stress

Risks in midlife	
Alcohol dependence and harmful use of alcohol	Shortened lifespan in general because of increased risk of heart disease, stroke, cancers, and liver cirrhosis, amnesia, cognitive deficits, sleep problems, peripheral neuropathy, gastrointestinal problems, decreased bone density and blood cell production
Smoking	Increases the risk of a range of cancers, heart disease and chronic obstructive pulmonary disease (COPD)
Smoking *and* drinking alcohol	Increases mortality rates significantly
Low levels of physical activity	Increases risk of cancer and heart disease
Excess weight in middle age	Degradation of the brain, increased risk of cancer, diabetes, heart diseases, vascular diseases, dementia, strokes, high blood pressure, mental illness, spending many years of life with a disability, as well as poorer social and economic conditions
Intimate relationship dissolutions and/or living alone	Greater risk of HIV, physical and mental health problems generally (depression and dementia specifically), higher mortality
Strained relationships with children	Depressive symptoms
Parenting grandchildren	Poorer physical health
Timing of the menopause	Early menopause is associated with an increased risk of osteoporosis and cardiovascular diseases whilst a later menopause is associated with increased risk of breast cancer
Early retirement	Higher mortality rates than those who retire at 65
Caring	Heart problems, arthritis and asthma. Caring may also impact negatively on personal and sexual relationships, employment opportunities, financial and social circumstances

course perspective also requires consideration of those factors that can threaten health and well-being as we progress through this final life stage. It is to these risks to health and well-being in older age that we now turn.

Discussion Point

To what extent do you think that health and well-being in old age are the 'cumulative risks of longstanding unhealthy habits' (Berger, 2011: 630)?

Risks and More Risks to Health and Well-Being in Old Age

Whilst there is inevitably some overlap in the risks to health and well-being in old age with those at other stages of the life course, there are several different ones that arise because of the nature of this life stage. Examples of these are retirement, deteriorating health and well-being, living arrangements and ageism. More significantly, the literature indicates that because of its length, the risks to health and well-being change, increase and accumulate from the beginning to the end of old age. We will therefore explore the main risks that have been identified and any changes in them that occur.

ACTIVITY 7.1

The grid set out below uses a different format from that used in other chapters because of the nature of this life stage. As you read through the rest of this section, try to identify any risks that are likely to increase during old age.

Risks that increase during old age

Lifestyle

Several aspects of older people's lifestyles threaten their health and well-being. For instance, there is evidence that there has been an increase in their alcohol consumption, particularly amongst women (McCormick et al., 2009; Emslie et al., 2011). This is a cause for concern for two reasons. We have already established that harmful drinking increases the risk of heart disease, stroke, cancers and liver cirrhosis, amnesia, cognitive deficits, sleep problems, peripheral neuropathy, gastrointestinal problems, decreased bone density and blood cell production. Harmful drinking in older people has further negative consequences because they are more sensitive to alcohol's negative health effects compared to younger adults and are more prone to fall injuries (Hallgren et al., 2010). Another aspect of older people's lifestyles that can be a threat to their health and well-being is weight control; those over 65 tend to have high rates of obesity and are less likely to address this risk to their health and well-being because older individuals tend to underestimate their own weight (Rayner et al., 2010; Peng Ng et al., 2011). On a more positive note, as Figure 7.1 shows, smoking prevalence in adults aged 60 and over has consistently been the lowest for all age groups during the last four decades. In addition, those who stop smoking between the ages of 60 and 75 years of age reduce their risk of dying prematurely by 50 per cent (Stegeman et al., 2012).

Physical inactivity in old age has been linked to increased mortality, 'cardiovascular disease, diabetes, obesity, osteoporosis, musculoskeletal problems, several cancers, depression and dementia' (Victor, 2010: 137). Although increasing numbers of older

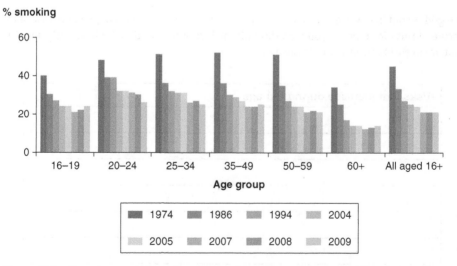

Figure 7.1 Prevalence of cigarette smoking by age, persons aged 16 and over, Great Britain, 1974–2009

Source: Cancer Research UK (2012).

people are engaging in moderate physical activity, levels decrease with advancing years (Green 2010; Stegeman et al., 2012). Similarly, other lifestyle factors in old age that are conducive to good health are often out of an individual's control. An example is sleep; good sleep is a prerequisite for older people's well-being and their ability to engage fully in daytime activities, yet advancing age is associated with progressive deterioration in the quality of sleep and increased sleep disturbance. If chronic sleep disturbance is untreated it 'degrades quality of later life, inhibits recovery and rehabilitation following illness, and is an independent risk factor for falls and depression' (SomnIA, 2010: 1) (SomnIA, 2010; Venn and Arber, 2011).

Retirement

In Chapter 6 we discussed some of the implications for health and well-being of early retirement. The average retirement age in the United Kingdom started to rise in the mid 1990s after falling for several decades. Although the age of retirement currently averages at 64.5 for men and 62.4 for women, 28 per cent of those over the retirement age and without a long-term illness of limitation are employed and some groups, such as professional people and those who are self-employed, work for longer (Berry, 2010; Economic and Social Research Council, 2011). Nevertheless, given increasing longevity, most people will spend at least a couple of decades of their life in retirement. It is therefore important to consider the short- and the long-term effects of retirement on the health and well-being of older people.

Some people find adjusting to life without paid work difficult and experience a loss of status and identity as well as isolation and loneliness. Recent findings show that alcohol consumption and weight increase post-retirement. Indeed, many employees who are in good health often want to work for longer but are not able to do so. However, whilst there is evidence that working on a flexible basis enhances health and well-being, there is a lack of evidence that retirement in itself harms health – it is when it coincides with low income and considerably reduced social contact that it can lead to higher morbidity and mortality rates in old age. With reference to low income, this is a particular issue for those who are retired. Until recently, there was a strong association between poverty and older age. Although policy initiatives helped poverty rates amongst the elderly to fall between 1997 and 2007, this fall has stalled in recent years and one in five people between the ages of 65 and 69 still live on a low income and this increases to one in three people for those aged 85 and over (McCormick et al., 2009; Berry, 2010; Burdorf, 2010; Norström and Palme, 2010; van Solinge and Henkens, 2010).

Moreover, some studies show that retirement has many positive effects in terms of substantial reductions in mental and physical fatigue and depressive symptoms. It also provides opportunities for those who have devoted considerable amounts of their time to paid work to pursue their own interests, socialise with friends and undertake volunteering. Although these sorts of activities have been found to enhance health and well-being, participation in them does drop 'significantly among people over 75' (McCormick et al., 2009: 9) (McCormick et al., 2009; Westerlund et al., 2010).

Deteriorating Health and Well-Being

Despite the potential benefits of being retired from paid employment as we saw in the previous section, physical and mental health generally tend to deteriorate throughout old age. For instance, disability rates increase in old age but particularly in those over the age of 80. Such deterioration often has a significant impact on quality of life and subjective well-being. Recent studies have shown that this increase in disability leads to worsening subjective well-being (Freedman et al., 2012). Deteriorating health can also be dramatic and have extremely negative outcomes. Using the example of dementia, as Figure 7.2 shows, the incidence of this condition rises sharply with age and is estimated to affect 25 per cent of those over 85. Dementia inevitably brings high levels of dependence for those who suffer from it (McCrone et al., 2008).

This deterioration in health and well-being in old age invariably has life-threatening consequences. Using the example of cancer to illustrate this, over a third (36 per cent) of all cancers are diagnosed in those over 75. Furthermore, as Figure 7.3 shows,

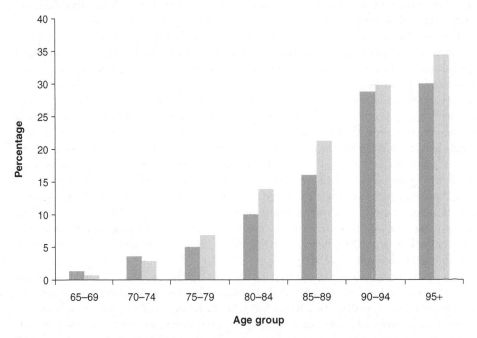

Figure 7.2   Prevalence of dementia in men and women over the age of 65

Source: McCrone et al. (2008: 112). Reproduced by permission of the King's Fund

Risks that increase during old age
Retirement: higher alcohol consumption and weight increase post-retirement
Low income and lack of social contact: both of these are associated with higher morbidity and mortality rates in old age. Those over 85 are more likely to be on a low income than those between the ages of 65 and 69. Hence, the risks posed by a low income to health and well-being are greater for those aged 85 plus
Reduction in activities that enhance health and well-being: this occurs among people over 75
Dementia: the incidence of this condition rises sharply with age and is estimated to affect 25 per cent of those over 85
Cancer: over a third (36 per cent) of all cancers are diagnosed in those over 75 and older. Death rates from cancer for both males and females rise with increasing age

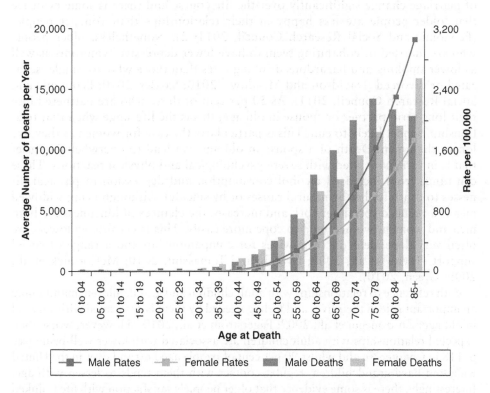

Figure 7.3 Average number of deaths per year and age-specific mortality rates for all cancers, United Kingdom, 2007–09

Source: Cancer Research UK (2011).

How are you doing with your grid? Here are some suggestions about points that you could have included so far.

death rates from cancer for both males and females rise with increasing age (Cancer Research UK, 2011).

Relationships

The most significant relationship for older people is usually that with their partner or spouse. Older men have to face possible loss of sexual potency that can reduce their self-esteem. In contrast, women have been found to find their old age to be a time of greater sexual freedom because their post-menopausal status means that they do not have to worry about contraception. The overall benefits of marriage change significantly over the life course and there is some evidence that 'older people are less happy in their relationships than younger people' (Economic and Social Research Council, 2011: 2). Nonetheless, older people who are married or cohabiting seem to have fewer depressive symptoms as well as lower smoking and hazardous drinking rates than those who are single, separated or divorced (Davidson and Meadows, 2010; Sassler, 2010; Economic and Social Research Council, 2011). As 50 per cent of those who are partnered lose their long-term partner or spouse in old age, this is the life stage when that relationship is most likely to end. This is particularly the case for women as they live longer than men. Death of a spouse in old age can lead to overwhelming grief that is in turn associated with severe psychological and physical reactions. These can range from increased alcohol consumption and depression to physical illnesses to death (either by natural causes or by suicide). Although being widowed means a reduced social network and increases the chances of loneliness for both men and women, women tend to cope more easily. This is because widowers are often very dependent on their wives for companionship and a range of social support (Taylor et al., 2008; Grundy and Tomassini, 2010; McCormick et al., 2009; Green, 2010).

With reference to relationships with adult children and grandchildren, maintaining an important role in their lives and feeling needed by them is associated with survival in old age (Zunzunegui et al., 2009; Fagerström et al., 2010). However, worse than expected relationships with adult children are associated with lower well-being (see p. 118 in Chapter 6), and whilst 90 per cent of people aged 60 and over in the United Kingdom have grandchildren, regular contact with them tends to lessen with age. Interestingly, there is some evidence that older people's satisfaction with life is linked more to the 'quality and quantity of their friendships than contact with younger family' (Green, 2010: 186) and that those who are childless are not necessarily less satisfied. However, the frequency of contact with friends declines after the age of 85, which indicates that people in late old age are more dependent on their family relationships for social contact and social support (Larkin, 2009; McCormick et al., 2009; Umberson et al., 2010).

Caring

Old age is often a time of taking on the role of carer to a spouse or partner. In addition, increased longevity means that many older people under 70 are caring for a parent (Pickard et al., 2007; McCormick et al., 2009). As we saw in Chapter 6 (see p. 121), caring has many negative impacts on health and well-being. Being a carer in old age can have further adverse consequences as a higher proportion of those at this life stage have a pre-existing condition that increases their vulnerability to the adverse effects of caring on health and well-being (Hanratty et al., 2007). In addition, as these carers are caring for those nearing the end of their life course, they are likely to have to undertake 'intensive caring', such as that involved in the later stages of dementia. This is known to increase levels of depression (McCrone et al., 2008; McCormick et al., 2009). Furthermore, caring for an elderly parent specifically has been shown to have adverse psychological effects not only on the carer but also on other members of the carer's family, for example spouses or partners (Amirkhanyan and Wolf, 2006). Finally, increasing numbers of grandparents over the age of 65 care for their grandchildren by either parenting them or providing childcare. This has a negative influence on the grandparents' own physical and mental health, particularly when carried out in combination with other caring roles (Glaser et al., 2006; Umberson, et al., 2010).

Living Arrangements

One of the consequences of demographic and political changes that have occurred during recent decades is that most older people now live in their own homes. Taking demographic changes first, there has been a decline in intergenerational households. One of the main reasons for this is geographical mobility that increases the chances of children moving away from their parents. Another reason is the higher incidence of marital breakdown; those parents who are not awarded custody may have weaker links with their children and therefore their risk of living alone in their old age is greater. As a result of the decline in intergenerational households, less than 5 per cent of the over 65s now live with an adult child (McCarthy and Thomas, 2004;

Vincent, 2006; Williams et al., 2007). In relation to political changes, the swing to community care and care at home within policy initiatives since the 1980s has meant that older people are able to live in their own homes and for longer. Hence, there has been a reduction of older people entering residential care (Baggott, 2004; Patsios, 2006).

Whilst living in their own homes in old age is what many older people prefer, it can adversely affect health and well-being, especially when they are in a single-person household. For instance, living in your own home can also mean spending between 70 to 90 per cent of your time alone and being at much greater risk of becoming socially isolated. This is particularly the case for older men and those in rural areas. Indeed, it is estimated that one-third of older people over the age of 65 years are lonely, with even higher rates among those aged over 85. Loneliness and social isolation are not only associated with increased vulnerability to depression, anxiety and poorer physical health but are also risk factors for mortality (Berkman et al., 2000; Department for Work and Pensions, 2005; Hauge and Kirkevold, 2012; Luo et al., 2012). Moreover, those older people living in single-person households 'are most likely to be living in non-decent homes' (McCormick et al., 2009: 6). This means that their houses can lack adequate heating, be damp, have infestation problems and be in a noisy neighbourhood. Thus, when older people live in their own homes there is a higher than average possibility of them living in poor-quality accommodation, which in turn poses further risks to their health and well-being (Larkin, 2011a).

Although fewer older people now live in residential establishments, a significant number of 'older' old people, especially those over 90, require some sort of residential care. Studies have found high levels of depression amongst those in residential homes and that fewer than half of them receive any form of treatment for this. Both treated and untreated depression, together with the lack of privacy, loss of independence, disempowerment and exclusion from everyday life that are inevitable consequences of living in such establishments have been cited as contributing to the fact that nearly half of older people die within 18 months of admission (McCormick et al., 2009; Larkin, 2011a).

Wherever older people live, there is a further major threat to their health and well-being – abuse. This can include sexual, physical, psychological or financial abuse and neglect. Whilst accurate statistics are difficult to obtain because elder abuse is often unreported, it is estimated that between 2 and 10 per cent of older people suffer some form of abuse. Perpetrators are usually partners, family members, neighbours and domiciliary care workers. Those aged 70 and over (particularly women over 70) are most vulnerable to abuse. However, those living in their own homes, especially those living on their own are even more vulnerable (Pritchard, 2006; Green, 2010).

Although these discussions have shown how older people's living arrangements can threaten their health and well-being, it is important not to romanticise the living arrangements of the elderly in the past. We need to remind ourselves that there is no ideal system, as every form of living arrangement for older people will have its drawbacks (Larkin, 2009).

Inadequate Healthcare

The way in which depression in older people living in residential care is often untreated was mentioned above. Indeed, many mental health problems amongst older people in general remain undiagnosed and untreated, more so than for other groups in the population (Allen, 2008). Using the example of depression once more, only a third of older people with depression ever discuss it with their GP and only half of them are diagnosed and treated, primarily with anti-depressants. With reference to older people suffering from dementia, fewer than half ever receive a diagnosis. The figure for older people in ethnic minority groups is even lower (Davison et al., 2007; Age Concern, 2008; Sharif, et al., 2008). In addition to depression and dementia, even higher numbers of older people experience unrecorded mental health problems such as alcohol use disorders and psychological distress because they are lonely, isolated or bereaved. The poor diagnosis and treatment rates of their mental health problems are sadly reflected in statistics that show that people between 55 and 74 have the highest rate of alcohol-related deaths in the United Kingdom, and older men and women have some of the highest suicide rates of all ages in the United Kingdom (Allen, 2008; Hallgren et al., 2010).

Such findings about the diagnosis and treatment of mental health problems in older people have been attributed to the use of insensitive diagnostic tools. Furthermore, many older people do not seek help because of the stigma of mental illness and their lack of awareness of its symptoms and a reluctance to talk about non-physical problems to their GP. There is also evidence that physical health problems are undiagnosed and untreated in older people. For instance, studies of cancer survival have revealed that older patients are under-treated and that their outcomes are poorer as a result. Factors identified as contributing to this are not only patient delay in presenting symptoms but also delays in primary care referral and the fact that they are less likely to receive intensive investigation and treatment (Foot and Harrison, 2011). More general obstacles to diagnosis and appropriate treatment for older people that have been identified are the continuation of age discrimination in healthcare (there are still age restrictions on screening and cardiac care) as well as **ageist** attitudes amongst some health professionals and also within the wider NHS (Age Concern, 2008; McCrone et al., 2008; Larkin, 2011a).

Other ways that have been identified in which healthcare can fail older people include the side effects of medication on them and the quality of care that they receive both in the community and in hospital. With reference to the former, medication can have more unpredictable effects on older people that in turn are a cause of morbidity and mortality. As we have talked about sleep disturbance in older people already, the research about hypnotic drugs prescribed for sleep problems will be used to illustrate this point. These drugs have been found to be associated with risks of impaired daytime functioning and falls when prescribed to older people. Amongst the very old they can exacerbate frailty and cognitive impairment (Thomson et al., 2010; Venn and Arber, 2011). In relation to the quality of healthcare for older people, studies have shown that there is inadequate out-of-hours provision for those at this life stage who are terminally ill, and the high number of those over 80 who die within 30 days of surgery has been blamed on the poor post-operative care that they receive (O'Brien and Jack 2010; Wilkinson et al., 2010).

Ageism and Discrimination

One of the reasons put forward above for the less than adequate healthcare that older people receive and the discrepancy between the numbers of those older

ACTIVITY 7.3

Here is a completed version of the grid that you were given in Activity 7.1. Compare the risks to health and well-being that increase during old age that you identified as you read through this section, with those on this grid.

Risks that increase during old age
Retirement: higher alcohol consumption and weight increase post-retirement
Low income and lack of social contact: both of these are associated with higher morbidity and mortality rates in old age. Those over 85 are more likely to be on a low income than those between the ages of 65 and 69. Hence, the risks posed by a low income to health and well-being are greater for those aged 85 plus
Reduction in activities that enhance health and well-being: this occurs among people over 75
Dementia: the incidence of this condition rises sharply with age and is estimated to affect 25 per cent of those over 85
Cancer: over a third (36 per cent) of all cancers are diagnosed in those over 75. Death rates from cancer for both males and females rise with increasing age
Frequency of contact with friends: this is linked to older people's satisfaction but declines after the age of 85

Risks that increase during old age
Loneliness and social isolation: one-third of older people over the age of 65 are lonely, and the rates among those aged over 85 are even higher. Loneliness and social isolation are associated with increased vulnerability to depression, anxiety and poorer physical health
Abuse (sexual, physical, psychological or financial abuse and neglect): those aged 70 and over (particularly women over 70) are most vulnerable to abuse
Inadequate healthcare: the high number of those over 80 who die within 30 days of surgery has been blamed on the poor post-operative care that they receive

people who want to work and those who actually do have some form of paid employment is ageism. Indeed, despite the passing of legislation, there is evidence that around a third of older people still experience age discrimination. Such discriminatory attitudes have been linked to negative images of old age and the way in which old age is culturally devalued (Social Exclusion Unit, 2005; Degnen, 2007; Green, 2010). As the high levels of discrimination on the grounds of advancing years can potentially threaten the health and well-being of older people, there have been many initiatives aimed at addressing this and improving practice (see below). There has also been a cultural shift over the past decade in attitudes to the elderly. This has been attributed in part to media attention to age discrimination and changes in advertising representations of older people; there has been a move from negative representations of them as being feeble and senile to more positive ones such as being healthy, fit, active and even sexual (Vincent, 2006; Williams et al., 2007).

Key Influences

In addition to showing how some of the risks to health and well-being in old age increase and accumulate as we progress through this life stage, the discussions above referred to other interacting factors that influence the outcomes of these risks. Gender was one of these factors and we saw how it can influence levels of alcohol consumption and social isolation. Various social and political changes were also mentioned. These included the decline in intergenerational households, the higher incidence of marital breakdown and the moves to community care and care at home. As we have seen throughout this book, the life course approach argues that the risks to health and well-being at each life stage interact with these sorts of factors as well as with the cumulative effects of risks in previous life stages. Furthermore, some of the more negative outcomes of these complex interactions can be offset by positive experiences over the life course that have 'protective effects' (Bryant et al., 2003: 363). This is illustrated by the way in which the relationship between childhood financial hardship and the higher incidence of illnesses in later life can be modified by higher earnings in young and middle adulthood (Tucker-Seeley et al., 2011). Thus, higher earnings in young and middle adulthood clearly have a 'protective effect' in old age. The way that retirement is beneficial in terms of reducing mental and physical fatigue and depressive symptoms is an example of a positive influence in old age itself. There is also evidence in the literature that personal qualities such as resilience reduce the risks to health and well-being associated with ageing (Doyle et al., 2010; Mertens, et al., 2011).

The variables identified as being the most influential at this stage come under the umbrella of the more general environmental, psychological, social, historical and biological influences that are deemed important at each life stage within the life course perspective. Hence, whilst the nature of their influence is specific to old age, there are similarities between these variables and those at other life stages.

Gender

There is a substantial body of evidence that gender shapes health and well-being in older age in several ways. Although women's employment patterns are changing, when compared to men they have spent fewer years in employment and experience both discontinuous employment and lower earnings. The relationship between lifetime earnings and pensions means that women are at a greater risk of living on a low income and in poverty in old age. Furthermore, as women spend a longer time in old age, they are more likely to see any income that they do have reduced, for example by healthcare expenses or running a single-person household. Low income in old age has been shown to lead to higher morbidity and mortality rates in old age. In contrast, older women tend to have a wider range of social networks that not only are sources of social support but can also protect against dementia and depression (McCormick et al., 2009; Norström and Palme, 2010; Platt, 2011).

Culture

Both culture and cultural changes can impact on old age in many different ways. First of all, certain aspects of a culture can have important implications. For instance, the United Kingdom has been found to be amongst Europe's worst countries for ageism (European Social Survey, 2011). Arguably, the threats posed to the health and well-being of older people in the United Kingdom discussed above are therefore greater than in other European countries. Another aspect of culture that has been found to be influential is the nature of family life; people who are part of a Mediterranean culture tend to be more involved in the lives of other members of their family. This involvement has been associated with survival in older people (Zunzunegui et al., 2009). The type of healthcare available in a country is also highly influential; there is evidence that it leads to differences in cancer survival rates as well as mortality rates for chronic illnesses in the elderly (McGauran, 2010; Foot and Harrison, 2011). With reference to social care, the quality of services for older people in the United Kingdom compares unfavourably with several other countries (Larkin, 2011a). In addition, the level of national investment in elder-focused technology plays a key role in determining older people's mobility, independence and quality of life (Joyce and Loe, 2010).

One of the most significant cultural changes in virtually all Western countries in the last few years has been the move to bring retirement ages more in line with increases in longevity by extending working life (Burdorf, 2010; van Solinge and Henkens, 2010). Another development within Westernised countries is the emphasis on eternal youth and the expansion of anti-ageing products and surgeries. There are many concerns about the health risks associated with this boom in anti-age therapies (Harris, 2010).

Socioeconomic Circumstances

The link between poorer socioeconomic circumstances and poorer health and well-being has frequently been referred to in this book. The same patterns can inevitably be observed in old age and there is even less chance of any weakening of the association because of the cumulative effects of having experienced a lifetime of disadvantage and more unhealthy lifestyles (Green, 2010; Rees Jones et al., 2011). Specific examples are the way in which frailty and health and social care utilisation have been found to be higher amongst those of lower socioeconomic status (Hoeck et al., 2011). In contrast, research has shown that those older people in higher socioeconomic groups are more likely to live longer in good health before retirement and expect to live longer post-retirement (Majer et al., 2011).

Ageing Well

What sorts of issues does the author of the following article argue need to be addressed in order to improve the lives of older people?

Who would want to grow old and reach a vintage age? A million pensioners live below the poverty line; more than a million aged 65 and older report that they are often or always lonely, chronic long-term conditions such as diabetes and heart disease plague

(Continued)

ACTIVITY 7.4

(Continued)

millions, public places make no concessions to the needs of the less agile while popular culture too often pushes anyone over 60 out of the frame unless he or she is attempting to pass as 20 years younger ... but we are on the threshold of a new era. We know much more about what can immunise us from the worst effects of ageing. Important elements are good health, a decent income and, perhaps most significant of all, robust relationships and connections to others. Genes and good fortune help but so will creating a different kind of society. One in which the growing gap between young and old is challenged; the value of experience is properly appreciated and success is no longer solely defined by what you earn and what you spend. ... In the US, for instance, organisations already exist that give truncated training to retirees who then take on an 'encore' career, in a different field from their first, often working to give something back to the community. ... Embracing rather than fighting against increased longevity also requires society to exercise a lot more imagination than it has hitherto shown. Lunch clubs, meals on wheels, old people's homes and sheltered accommodation are all concepts born of their time, but desperately in need of an update. Likewise, the curse of our age – isolation – also requires a more proactive attempt at a cure. An older person may begin adult life with friends; have his or her circle expand with a partnership, but then find that those ties are severed by death or divorce or circumstance. So how do you forge new bonds in your seventies or eighties? (Roberts, 2011)

As you read through the rest of this section, think about the extent to which current policy initiatives are directed at the issues identified in the article.

For over a decade there has been an emphasis in national and international health and well-being policies on 'successful ageing' and 'active ageing'. Indeed, this emphasis is reflected in the fact that 2012 was designated as the European Year for Active Ageing in order to increase the profile of older citizens within Europe. The overarching theme within these policies is the promotion of the health and well-being of older people by addressing different aspects of their lives. For instance, many initiatives have aimed to ensure that older people maintain their independence, enjoy an active leisure lifestyle, engage with life and society in order to reduce their social isolation, have an adequate income and are provided with education and learning opportunities. Some have also focused on tackling ageism and discrimination, protecting older people from abuse and treating them with dignity. Others have introduced measures in order to ensure that they receive high-quality support and healthcare throughout their old age, including at the end of their lives (World Health Organization, 2002; Department of Health, 2008; McCormick et al., 2009; Royal College of Psychiatrists, 2010; Cattan et al., 2011). There has also been a considerable amount of research into factors that contribute to 'successful ageing' and 'active ageing' around identifying ways of using the pension system to incentivise gradual retirement options, the use of technological tools to help older people to sustain their health and well-being, and improving the sleep patterns in those older people who experience poor sleep (Berry, 2010; SomnIA, 2010; EuroHealthNet, 2012).

A life course perspective features strongly in the approaches being adopted. Examples include the drive to 'encourage young adults to prepare for old age in their health, social and financial practices' (World Health Organization, 2002: 52), to increase opportunities for people during the course of their working lives in order to accrue more pension rights, and interventions to promote healthy lifestyles and mental health across the whole life course (ibid.; Royal College of Psychiatrists, 2010; EuroHealthNet, 2011; Knapp et al., 2011).

Any policies addressing the needs of older people are plagued by problems of obtaining a reliable information base. This is particularly the case for those policies that focus on people aged 85 and over. As those in this age group are more likely to suffer from some degree of cognitive impairment, research about them tends to use family and other key gatekeepers. Reliance on such intermediaries can compromise the accuracy of the findings (Davies et al., 2010). The political mainstreaming of 'successful ageing' and 'active ageing' has also been criticised for being socially exclusive. Examples are the way in which the needs of the growing number of older people from ethnic minority groups are overlooked and how some aspects of 'active ageing' (such as active leisure activities) appear to be the province of those who are culturally and materially advantaged. Therefore, it is the White, healthy, educated, upper-class and middle-class people who are more likely to engage with such initiatives (Chatzitheochari and Arber, 2011; Patel, 2012). In addition, policies that emphasise 'successful ageing' and 'active ageing' have been accused of presenting ageing as a 'problem' that must be 'managed' and using negative political rhetoric about the social burden of ageing in relation to the pressure on the National Health Service, the cost of pensions and social care. In so doing, they overlook not only older people's individuality and the complexity of their strategies for actively managing their lives, but also what they do to contribute to society in terms of the social cohesion of society by providing support to their peers and to younger generations (Powell et al., 2007). Consequently, critics argue that we need to move away from a:

> ... one-size-fits-all policy approaches that treat older people as if they are all alike are alienating and inappropriate. Instead, older people need inclusive policy approaches that enable them to live their lives on their own terms. To ensure that older people are actively engaged, policy makers should stop emphasising the costs posed by an ageing population and start building on the many positive contributions that older people already make to our society. (Bazalgette et al., 2011: 9)

Discussion Point

Is it realistic to think that ageing can be 'successful' or 'active'?

Conclusions

This chapter has covered a wide range of issues in relation to a life course analysis of health and well-being in old age; it has presented evidence about the potential outcomes of cumulative risks and experiences from conception, through to infancy, childhood, adolescence, young adulthood and middle adulthood. In addition, it has also shown how the risks to health and well-being change, increase and accumulate from the beginning to the end of old age. Therefore, it can be concluded that risks to health and well-being do accumulate across the whole life course. As argued in other chapters, on the basis of the existing research it is not possible to ascertain whether particular life stages are more significant than others in influencing 'an individual's health and well-being across their whole life' (Graham, 2009: 26). Nonetheless, both the sheer length of old age and increasing longevity render this a highly significant life stage – arguments in themselves for further investment in measures throughout the life course that both ensure optimum health and well-being when we reach old age and maintain our health and well-being throughout this life stage.

Summary

- The irreversible physical and cognitive changes that characterise old age are often accompanied by a deterioration in health and well-being throughout this life stage
- Whilst the effects of cumulative risks from all of the preceding life stages contribute to poorer health and well-being, these risks can be mediated by a number of interacting variables, some of which have 'protective effects'. Influences on the risks to our health and well-being identified in the preceding life stages are parental influences, poverty and social disadvantage, culture, gender, the economy and personality
- Risks to health and well-being during old age tend to increase and accumulate. The main risks are lifestyle factors (such as alcohol consumption, weight control, physical inactivity and sleep), retirement, deteriorating health and well-being, relationships, caring, living arrangements, healthcare and ageism
- Influences on these risks to health and well-being during old age are gender, culture and socioeconomic circumstances
- 'Successful ageing' and 'active ageing' have become the focus of national and international health and well-being policies. As a result, there has been an emphasis on the maintenance and promotion of the health and well-being of older people by improving many different aspects of their lives

Further Study

Lifespan books have chapters dedicated to old age that have good overviews of changes that occur at this life stage. Examples are K. Berger, *The Developing Person through the Lifespan*, 8th edn (New York: Worth Publishers, 2011); and D. Boyd and H. Bee, *Lifespan Development* (Upper Saddle River, NJ: Pearson, 2012). Chapters 2 to 5 in C. Victor, *Ageing, Health and Care* (Bristol: Policy Press, 2010), have some very useful information about the risks to health and well-being in old age. J. Allen, *Older People and Well-Being* (London: Institute for Public Policy Research, 2008), provides an interesting analysis of how some of the key social trends impact on older people and their well-being. Journals such as *Ageing and Society* are good sources if you want to read about recent research. To keep up with policy initiatives about healthy ageing visit: www.healthyageing.eu

Postscript

The unique synthesis of the existing body of national and international literature on health and well-being across all the life stages undertaken in this book from a life course perspective provides the most comprehensive account of health and well-being from a life course perspective that exists to date. Furthermore, it unequivocally supports the main argument put forward within the life course approach that risks to health and well-being accumulate across the whole life course – from conception, through to infancy, childhood, adolescence, adulthood and old age. Other aspects of the life course perspective that were endorsed were its emphasis on the importance of other influences in each life stage of the life course and the way that positive experiences over the life course can offset exposure to negative events and risk factors.

However, there was little support for the emphasis placed by those who adopt an epidemiological approach on the importance of the timing of exposure to events in our lives determining their eventual impact on our health and well-being. Similarly, Graham's assertion that 'pregnancy, childhood and adolescence' are more significant in terms of 'an individual's health and well-being across their whole life' (Graham, 2009: 26) remained unproven. As pointed out in Chapter 1, identifying all the processes that can affect our health and well-being throughout our lives raises 'formidable methodological challenges' (Graham, 2007: 145). Moreover, research in this area is rapidly gathering momentum and capturing the latest findings can be problematic even for the most enthusiastic researchers. Therefore the lack of corroboration of some aspects of the life course approach to health and well-being does not detract from its value in understanding the patterning of health and illness over the life course and its subsequent role in the contemporary public health movement. Nonetheless it does highlight areas which need further research in order to develop the strengths of the life course approach more generally. In addition, research for this book foregrounded other national and international developments that will need to be considered in future theoretical models of life course processes; at the time of writing, we are in the middle of a global recession. Serious concerns are being raised about the implications for health and well-being of issues such as rising poverty levels amongst children and working-age poverty (Brewer et al., 2012). Examples of other matters high on the global agenda are widening health inequalities, the incidence of chronic diseases and the world-wide obesity pandemic (Busse et al., 2010; Marmot, 2010; Swinburn et al., 2011). Therefore, whilst the life course approach currently provides us with invaluable insights, it does require ongoing targeted research and needs to respond to local, national and global changes in order to maximise its contributions to the understanding of health and well-being and the development of effective policies.

Glossary

Acquired Immune Deficiency Syndrome (AIDS): caused by the Human Immunodeficiency Virus, it results in the progressive failure of the immune system. This in turn leads to life-threatening infections and cancers. As yet, there is no known cure

acute illness: a short-term illness, such as a sickness bug or a chest infection

ageism: when a person is discriminated against on the grounds of age

age-related macular degeneration (AMD): an eye disease that involves deterioration of the retina. It mainly affects the elderly and is hard to treat. Whilst it eventually leads to legal blindness, individuals affected are not completely sightless

Alzheimer's disease: this is the most common form of dementia (see below) and is characterised by gradual deterioration of memory and personality

anorexia nervosa: an eating disorder that means that sufferers have a morbid fear of gaining weight. Their body image is distorted, with the result that they dramatically restrict their eating, lose significant amounts of weight and for females menstruation ceases

attention deficit hyperactivity disorder (ADHD): often referred to as ADHD, this is a group of behavioural symptoms that include inattentiveness, hyperactivity and impulsiveness. Common symptoms include a short attention span, restlessness, being easily distracted and constant fidgeting. Many people with ADHD also have additional problems, such as sleep disorders or learning difficulties

binge drinking: the purposeful consumption of alcohol over a short period of time with the primary intention of becoming intoxicated. It is more common in males during adolescence and young adulthood

biomedical approach to health: this rests on an assumption that all causes of disease (both mental disorders and physical disease) can be understood in biological terms. It also views disease and sickness as deviations from normal functioning that medicine has the power to put right with its scientific knowledge and understanding of the human body

blood pressure: the pressure exerted by circulating blood on the walls of blood vessels. Although average values for this pressure have been computed with their relevance to general health, there is often a large variation from person to person and it also varies in individuals from moment to moment

body mass index (BMI):   often referred to as BMI, this is a measurement of a person's weight in kilograms divided by their height in metres squared

bulimia nervosa: an eating disorder involving frequent compulsions to eat large quantities of food over a relatively short period of time. These episodes of binge eating are preceded by intense feelings of anxiety and tension and often end with self-induced vomiting and/or excessive use of laxatives

cataracts: this is an eye disease that is common amongst the elderly and involves a thickening of the lens in the eye with the result that vision becomes cloudy and distorted

chronic illness: a long-term health disorder that interferes with social interaction and role performance. Examples are multiple sclerosis, arthritis and Alzheimer's disease

conduct disorders: these are recognised psychiatric conditions and involve persistent disobedience and defiance. Typical behaviours are frequent and severe temper tantrums (beyond the usual age for these), excessive levels of fighting and bullying, cruelty to others and to animals, criminal activities and running away from home

congenital heart defect (CHD):   this is a defect in the heart that is present at birth and can obstruct blood flow in the heart or vessels near it, cause blood to flow through the heart in an abnormal pattern or affect the heart's rhythm. Some defects go undetected throughout life but symptoms of CHDs in childhood are shortness of breath, underdeveloping of limbs and muscles, skin discolouration, poor feeding or growth and respiratory infections

dementia: the irreversible loss of brain functioning caused by brain damage or disease. It becomes more common with age and leads to impaired judgement, memory and problem-solving ability. The main types of dementia are Alzheimer's disease, vascular dementia, fronto-temporal dementia, dementia with Lewy bodies and mixed dementia

discourse: groups of ideas or patterned ways of thinking that shape the understanding about a particular subject in society. Use of language is central to the construction of discourses. A variety of discourses can exist at any one time; some discourses are more powerful than others and often reflect the interests of dominant and/or political groups

discrimination: when members of a particular group in society are denied resources, rewards and opportunities that are available to and can be obtained by others in society

dysporia: a medically recognised transient psychological condition in which a person experiences intense feelings of sadness, sorrow and anguish, anxiety and discontent. It is also accompanied by irritability and indifference to the world

empty nest syndrome: refers to the negative reactions that parents experience when their children leave the parental home and the difficulties that they have in making the adjustments required. However, some parents enjoy their newfound sense of freedom

encephalopathy: injury to the brain that may cause irreversible damage to the brain, resulting in a variety of brain disorders such as loss of cognitive function, seizures and respiratory abnormalities

epidemiology: the study of patterns of disease within a population over time. It involves statistical measures to establish the risk factors of diseases as well as their social origins and transmission

exercise referral schemes: these aim to identify inactive adults in the primary care setting. They involve referral to a third-party service that takes responsibility for prescribing and monitoring an exercise programme tailored to the needs of individual patients

externalising behaviour problems: childhood behaviour problems that are manifested in outward behaviour and reflect the child negatively acting on the *external* environment. Examples are disruptive, hyperactive and aggressive behaviours. Studies show that childhood externalising behaviour problems are strong predictors of adult crime and violence

Female Athlete Triad (FAT):   this is most common amongst young women who take part in sports that emphasise low body weight (for example, ballet dancing and ice-skating) and is the physical manifestation of the pathological pursuit of exercise regimes. It is often coupled with an inappropriate diet

Fetal Alcohol Spectrum Disorders (FASD):   these occur because of the way that alcohol damages fetal brain development and the central nervous system. This damage can result in facial deformities, physical and emotional developmental problems, memory and attention deficits, as well as cognitive and behavioural problems

gestational diabetes: high blood glucose (hyperglycaemia) during pregnancy. In most cases it can be controlled through diet and exercise and does not continue beyond pregnancy. However, women with gestational diabetes are at increased risk of developing Type 2 diabetes mellitus in later life

glaucoma: an eye disease that involves pressure resulting from a buildup of fluid within the eye which causes damage to the optic nerve. It can be successfully treated but if left untreated it can destroy vision

health-related quality of life: a broad, multidimensional concept that encompasses physical and mental health, social and role functioning and general well-being.

Human Immunodeficiency Virus (HIV): a virus that causes Acquired Immune Deficiency Syndrome (AIDS). The latter is a condition that results in the progressive failure of the immune system that in turn leads to life-threatening infections and cancers. HIV infections can be transferred during unsafe sex, use of contaminated needles, through breast milk and from an infected mother to her baby at birth. Although HIV is still incurable, treatment with antiretroviral drugs usually reduces both the mortality and the morbidity of those infected with the virus

hypertension: this is also known as high blood pressure and occurs when the heart has to work harder than it should to pump the blood around the body. This puts a strain on the arteries and the heart and persistent hypertension is one of the risk factors for stroke, myocardial infarction, heart failure, arterial aneurysm and chronic kidney failure. Moderate hypertension can also shorten life expectancy. Although dietary and lifestyle changes can improve blood pressure control and decrease the risk of associated health complications, drug treatment is often necessary for patients for whom lifestyle changes prove ineffective or insufficient

in utero: this literally means 'in the uterus'. It has different meanings in different contexts; in biology, the phrase is used to describe the state of an embryo or fetus. In legal contexts, it is used to refer to unborn children

ischaemic heart disease: a disease characterised by reduced blood supply to the heart muscle. Symptoms include chest pain on exertion and decreased exercise tolerance. It is a major cause of hospital admissions and the most common cause of death in most Western countries

lone parent family: usually defined as a divorced, separated, single or widowed mother or father living without a spouse (and not cohabiting) with his or her never-married dependent child or children

low birth weight: this refers to a baby who weighs less than 2500 grams (5 lbs) at birth

menarche: the beginning of a woman's reproductive life that coincides with the onset of menstruation

menopause: typically occurs in women between the ages of 42–58 and is officially defined as being reached a year after a woman's last period. It involves a set of changes over a number of years: the ovaries slowly produce less oestrogen and progesterone, which leads to irregular menstruation and its eventual complete cessation. Menopausal symptoms include vaginal dryness, night sweats, hot flushes, increased stress, breast tenderness, forgetfulness and mood changes. Women are at a much higher risk of osteoporosis after the menopause as lowered oestrogen levels lead to bone loss

morbidity rates: the number and patterns of physical and mental illnesses within a designated group at a given time, expressed as a rate per 100,000 of the population

mortality rates: the number and causes of deaths within a designated group at a given time, expressed as a rate per 100,000 of the population

mother–child attachment: the bond between a mother and child. This requires continuity and sensitivity in care-giving from babyhood, and plays an important role in a child's future development in general but particularly in their mental health

neuroendocrine systems: the interactions that take place between the nervous system and the endocrine system that control essential physiological functions such as reproduction in all of its aspects, metabolism, blood pressure and the body's response to stress and infection

non-accidental injury: the deliberate physical or psychological/emotional mistreatment or neglect of a vulnerable person, such as a child or an old person, that results in harm, potential for harm or threat of harm to that person

obesity: a level of body fat that is harmful. A person is considered obese if they have a Body Mass Index (BMI) of 30 or more

obsessive compulsive disorder (OCD): an anxiety disorder characterised by recurrent urges to repeat certain behaviours or avoid certain situations. Examples are repeated checking and excessive washing or cleaning

overweight: this involves an excess of body fat and having a Body Mass Index (BMI) of 25 or more

perinatal asphyxia: this is the medical condition resulting from deprivation of oxygen during labour. It can lead to brain damage and long-term physical and cognitive impairment

poor fetal growth: definitions are controversial and there are many influences on fetal growth. Poor fetal growth is most commonly said to be occurring when a fetus is small for its gestational age

pre-eclampsia: affects 2 to 5 per cent of pregnancies. It is usually diagnosed from around 20 weeks and is most common in the third trimester of pregnancy. There are usually no symptoms apart from protein in the urine and a high blood pressure reading. If untreated, pre-eclampsia can have serious consequence for the mother and her unborn child

pregnancy trimesters: pregnancy is typically broken into three trimesters to describe the changes that take place. Each trimester is about three months: the first trimester is weeks 1 to 12, the second is weeks 13 to 27, and the third is weeks 28 to 42

presbycusis: age-related hearing loss that affects around 40 per cent of those over 65

preterm birth: refers to the birth of a baby at less than 37 weeks gestation. Births at less than 32 weeks gestation are known as 'very preterm births' whilst those between 32 and 36 weeks gestation are called 'moderately preterm birth'

psychopathology: a generic term used to describe mental illness, mental distress and abnormal/maladaptive behaviour

public health: this movement aims to improve lives by reducing inequalities in the incidence of ill health and diseases (such as heart disease and mental illness) at population and community level, rather than at an individual level. The focus of public health intervention is the prevention of health problems and identifying illness at a stage where treatment is more likely to be effective. It makes extensive use of the life course approach to track the causes, progression and pattern of health problems in order to identify the most effective ways of preventing them from developing at different life stages

puerperal psychoses: also known as postpartum psychoses and refers to a group of mental illnesses that start suddenly following childbirth. Some patients have manic symptoms, such as euphoria, hyperactivity, irritability, violence and grandiose delusions. Others have severe depression, with delusions, verbal hallucinations and stupor. There are also those who switch from mania to depression (or vice versa) within the same episode

reconstituted family: a household unit including a stepparent as a consequence of divorce, separation and remarriage. This type of family is created when a new partnership is formed by a mother and/or father who already have dependent children. Since most children remain with their mother following divorce or separation, stepfamilies are more likely to have a stepfather than a stepmother

sexually transmitted diseases (STDs):   these are illnesses that are usually transmitted between humans by means of human sexual behaviour, including vaginal intercourse, oral sex and anal sex. Some STDs can also be transmitted via the use of intravenous (IV) drug needles after their use by an infected person, as well as through childbirth or breastfeeding. Examples are chlamydia, gonorrhea and genital warts. STDs are also known as sexually transmitted infections (STIs)

social construction: this refers to the way that aspects of society or behaviour are 'constructed' in a particular way as a result of social relations and human agency rather than being 'natural' or biological in origin. Social constructions vary histori-cally, socially and culturally and are therefore essentially contestable

social support: this is provided by positive involvement in social networks. It has been shown to act as a buffer to stress and mental ill health, particularly if intimate and confiding relationships are involved

status inconsistency: where someone ranks high on one status indicator, such as education, but low on another, such as occupation or income

substance use disorder: the pathological overindulgence in and dependence on a non-medical drug or other chemical. This disorder has detrimental effects on physi-cal and mental health as well as having adverse social consequences, such as failure to meet school, work and family commitments, interpersonal conflicts and legal problems

suicidal ideation: a term for thoughts about suicide, which may involve a detailed plan. Whilst most people who engage in suicidal ideation do not commit suicide, some do go on to attempt suicide

teenage birth rate: the number of births per 1000 women aged 15 to 19

Type 1 diabetes: this occurs when the body does not produce any insulin at all and involves insulin injections for life. It is therefore often referred to as insulin-dependent diabetes. Those with Type 1 diabetes also have to make sure that their blood glucose levels stay balanced by eating a healthy diet and carrying out regular blood tests

Type 2 diabetes: this is far more common than Type 1 diabetes and is often associ-ated with obesity. It occurs when not enough insulin is produced by the body for it to function properly, or when the body's cells do not react to insulin. Those with Type 2 diabetes are usually able to control their symptoms by eating a healthy diet and monitoring their blood glucose level. However, as Type 2 diabetes is a progres-sive condition, they may eventually need to take insulin medication, usually in the form of tablets

venous thrombosis: a blood clot in the vein is called a venous thrombosis, and an example of this is deep vein thrombosis (DVT) when a blood clot occurs in a deep vein, usually in the leg. The usual symptoms of deep vein thrombosis include pain, tenderness, swelling of the leg and possible discolouration. If the thrombosis is in the thigh veins the whole leg may be swollen

vital organs: these are the cardiovascular, respiratory, digestive, lymphatic and renal/urinary organs. They are *vital* to the human body because they work together to do necessary jobs needed for our survival

References

Abebe, D.S., Lien, L., Torgersen, L. and von Soest, T. (2012) 'Binge eating, purging and non-purging compensatory behaviours decrease from adolescence to adulthood: a population-based, longitudinal study', *BMC Public Health*, 12: 32.

Age Concern (2008) *Undiagnosed, Untreated, At Risk: The Experiences of Older People with Depression*. London: Age Concern England.

Aiyama, H., Utsunomiya, A., Suzuki, S., Hirano, T., Suzuki, I., Nimura, T., Nishino, A. and Sakurai, Y. (2009) 'A case of enlargement of an intradiploic epidermoid cyst by a head contusion', *Brain and Nerve*, 61 (6): 707–10.

Alcorn, K.L., O'Donovan, A., Patrick, J.C., Creedy, D., Devilly, G.J. (2010) 'A prospective longitudinal study of the prevalence of post-traumatic stress disorder resulting from childbirth events', *Psychological Medicine*, 40 (11): 1849–59.

Aliyu, M.H., O'Neill, L., Beloglovvkin, V., Zoorab, R. and Salihu, H.M. (2010) 'Maternal alcohol use and medically indicated vs. spontaneous preterm birth outcomes: a population-based study', *European Journal of Public Health*, 20 (5): 582–7.

Allen, J. (2008) *Older People and Well-Being*. London: Institute for Public Policy Research.

Allen, P. (2011) 'France's young binge drinkers upset cafe society with their "British boozing"', *Observer*, 24 July, p. 25.

Almquist, Y.M. (2011) 'Childhood friendships and adult health: findings from the Aberdeen children of the 1950s Cohort study', *European Journal of Public Health*, 22 (3): 378–83.

Alwan, N., Siddiqi, K., Thomson, H. and Cameron, I. (2010) 'Children's exposure to second-hand smoke in the home: a household survey in the North of England', *Health and Social Care in the Community*, 18 (3): 257–63.

Amato, R.R. (2010) 'Research on divorce: continuing trends and new developments', *Journal of Marriage and Family*, 72 (3): 650–66.

Amirkhanyan, A.A. and Wolf, D.A. (2006) 'Parent care and the stress process: findings from panel data', *Journals of Gerontology, Series B: Psychological Sciences and Social Sciences*, 61 (5): S248–55.

Anokye, N.K., Trueman, P., Green, C., Pavey, T.G., Hillsdon, M. and Taylor, R.S. (2011) 'The cost-effectiveness of exercise referral schemes', *BMC Public Health*, 11: 954.

Appel, L.J. (2005). 'Hypertension: dietary factors', *Journal of Animal Physiology and Animal Nutrition*, 89 (11): 433–50.

Arber, S. and Ginn, J. (1995) *Connecting Gender and Ageing: A Sociological Approach*. Buckingham: Oxford University Press.

Aries, P. (1965) *Centuries of Childhood*. London: Cape.

Arksey, H., Kemp, P., Glendinning, C., Kotchetkova, I. and Toze, R. (2005) *Carers' Aspirations and Decisions Around Work and Retirement*. Leeds: Department for Work and Pensions.

Asthana, A. (2010) 'Parents find a new freedom after children leave the nest', *Observer*, 8 August, p. 15.

Atkinson, A., Elliott, G., Bellis, M. and Sumnall, H. (2011) *Young People, Alcohol and the Media*. York: Joseph Rowntree Foundation.

Baggott, R. (2004) *Health and Health Care in Britain*, 3rd edn. Basingstoke: Macmillan.

Balsa, A.I., Giuliano, L.M. and French, M.T. (2011) 'The effects of alcohol use on academic achievement in high school', *Economics of Education Review*, 30 (1): 1–15.

Ban, L., Gibson, J.E., West, J. and Tata, L.J. (2010) 'Association between perinatal depression in mothers and the risk of childhood infections in offspring', *BMC Public Health*, 10: 799.

Barlow, J. and Svanberg, P.O. (eds) (2010) *Keeping the Baby in Mind*. London: Routledge.

Bartlett, J., Grist, M. and Hahn, B. (2011) *Under the Influence*. London: Demos.

Bartley, M., Blane, D. and Montgomery, S. (1997) 'Health and the life course: why safety nets matter', *British Medical Journal*, 314 (7088): 1194–6.

Batty, G.D., Lewars, H., Emslie, C., Benzeval, M. and Hunt, K. (2008) 'Problem drinking and exceeding guidelines for "sensible" alcohol consumption in Scottish men: associations with life course socioeconomic disadvantage in a population-based cohort study', *BMC Public Health*, 8: 302.

Bazalgette, L., Tew, P., Holden, J., Hubble, N. and Morrison, J. (2011) *Ageing is not a Policy Problem to be Solved: Coming of Age*. London: Demos.

Beauchamp, A., Wolfe, R., Magliano, D., Turrell, G., Tonkin, A., Shaw, J. and Peeters, A. (2011) 'Incidence of cardiovascular risk factors by education level 2000–2005: the Australian diabetes, obesity, and lifestyle (AusDiab) cohort study', *Longitudinal and Life Course Studies*, 2 (3): 331–45.

Beckett, C. (2009) *Human Growth and Development*, 7th edn. London: Sage.

Ben-Shlomo, Y. and Kuh, D. (2002) 'A life course approach to chronic disease epidemiology: conceptual models, empirical challenges and interdisciplinary perspectives', *International Journal of Epidemiology*, 31 (2): 285–93.

Bendelow, G. (2009) *Health, Emotion and the Body*. Cambridge: Polity Press.

Benzies, K.M., Trute, B., Worthington, C., Reddon, J., Keown, L.-A. and Moore, M. (2011) 'Assessing psychological well-being in mothers of children with disability: evaluation of the parenting morale index and family impact of childhood disability scale', *Journal of Pediatric Psychology*, 36 (5): 506–16.

Beresford, B., Sloper, T. and Bradshaw, J. (2005) 'Physical health', in J. Bradshaw and E. Mayhew (eds), *The Well-Being of Children in the UK*, 2nd edn. London: Save the Children Fund.

Berger, K. (2011) *The Developing Person through the Lifespan*, 8th edn. New York: Worth Publishers.

Berkman, L.F., Glass, T., Brissette, I. and Sutman, T.E. (2000) 'From social integration to health: Durkheim in the new millennium', *Social Science and Medicine*, 51: 843–57.

Berry, C. (2010) *The Future of Retirement*. London: International Longevity Centre.

Biddle, L., Donovan, J., Hawton, K., Kapur, N. and Gunnell, D. (2008) 'Suicide and the Internet', *British Medical Journal*, 336: 800–2.

Blackwell, D.L., Hayward, M.D. and Crimmins, E.M. (2001) 'Does childhood health affect chronic morbidity in later life?', *Social Science and Medicine*, 52 (8): 1269–84.

Blanchflower, D.G. and Oswald, A.J. (2008) 'Is well-being U-shaped over the life cycle?', *Social Science and Medicine*, 66 (8): 1733–49.

Boardman, J.D. and Alexander, K.B. (2011) 'Stress trajectories, health behaviors, and the mental health of Black and White young adults', *Social Science and Medicine*, 72 (10): 1659–66.

Boffey, D. (2011) 'Growing up gets tougher for girls as "teen angst" levels rise', *Observer*, 17 April, p. 15.

Boone-Heinonen, J., Diez Roux, A.V., Kiefe, C.I., Lewis, C.E., Guilkey, D.K. and Gordon-Larsen, P. (2011) 'Neighborhood socioeconomic status predictors of physical activity through young to middle adulthood: the CARDIA study', *Social Science and Medicine*, 72 (5): 641–9.

Borgonovi, F. (2010) 'A life cycle approach to the analysis of the relationship between social capital and health in Britain', *Social Science and Medicine*, 71 (11): 1927–34.

Bowlby, J. (1965) *Child Care and the Growth of Love*. Harmondsworth: Penguin Books.

Boyd, D. and Bee, H. (2012) *Lifespan Development*. Upper Saddle River, NJ: Pearson.

Bracke, P.F., Colman, E., Symoens, S.A. and van Praag, L. (2010) 'Divorce, divorce rates, and professional care seeking for mental health problems in Europe: a cross-sectional population-based study', *BMC Public Health*, 10: 224.

Bradshaw, J. and Mayhew, E. (eds) (2005) *The Well-Being of Children in the UK*, 2nd edn. London: Save the Children Fund.

Bradshaw, J., Hoelscher, P. and Richardson, D. (2006) *Comparing Child Well-Being in OECD Countries: Concepts and Methods*. Florence: United Nations Children's Fund (UNICEF).

Braig, S., Peter, R., Nagel, G., Hermann, S., Rohrmann, S. and Linseisen, J. (2011) 'The impact of social status inconsistency on cardiovascular risk factors, myocardial infarction and stroke in the EPIC-Heidelberg cohort', *BMC Public Health*, 11: 104.

Brandlistuen, R.E., Stene-Larsen, K., Holmstrøm, H., Landolt, M.A., Eskedal, L.T. and Vollrath, M.E. (2011) 'Symptoms of communication and social impairment in toddlers with congenital heart defects', *Child: Care, Health and Development*, 37 (1): 37–43.

Brekke, M. and Straand, J. (2011) 'Does present use of cardiovascular medication reflect elevated cardiovascular risk scores estimated ten years ago? A population-based longitudinal observational study', *BMC Public Health*, 11: 144.

Brennan, P.L., Schutte, K.K., Moos, B.S. and Moos, R.H. (2011) 'Twenty-year alcohol-consumption and drinking-problem trajectories of older men and women', *Journal of Studies on Alcohol and Drugs*, 72 (2): 308–21.

Brewer, M., Browne, J. and Joyce, R. (2012) *Child and Working-Age Poverty from 2010 to 2020*. London: Institute for Fiscal Studies.

Brewer, M., Browne, J. and Sutherland, H. (2006) *What Will it Take to End Child Poverty?* York: Joseph Rowntree Foundation.

British Medical Association Board of Science (2007) *Fetal Alcohol Spectrum Disorders: A Guide for Healthcare Professionals*. London: British Medical Association.

Brixval, C.S., Rayce, S.L.B., Rasmussen, M., Holstein, B.E. and Due, P. (2011) 'Overweight, body image and bullying: an epidemiological study of 11- to 15-years olds', *European Journal of Public Health*, 21 (1): 122–8.

Broekhuizen, K.M., van Poppel, M.N.M., Lando, L.J., Koppes, L.J.K., Brug, J. and van Mechelen, W. (2010) 'A tailored lifestyle intervention to reduce the cardiovascular disease risk of individuals with Familial Hypercholesterolemia (FH): design of the PRO-FIT randomised controlled trial', *BMC Public Health*, 10: 69.

Brouwers, E.P.M., van Baa, A.L. and Pop, V.J.M. (2001) 'Maternal anxiety during pregnancy and subsequent infant development', *Infant Behavior and Development*, 24 (1): 95–106.

Brown, A.E., Raynor, P., Benton, D. and Lee, M.D. (2010a) 'Indices of Multiple Deprivation predict breastfeeding duration in England and Wales', *European Journal of Public Health*, 20 (2): 231–5.

Brown, D., Anda, R.F., Felitti, V.J., Edwards, V.J., Malarcher, A.M., Croft, J.B. and Giles, W.H. (2010b) 'Adverse childhood experiences are associated with the risk of lung cancer: a prospective cohort study', *BMC Public Health*, 10: 20.

Brown, J.E., Broom, D.H., Nicholson, J.M. and Bittman, M. (2010c) 'Do working mothers raise couch potato kids? Maternal employment and children's lifestyle behaviours and weight in early childhood', *Social Science and Medicine*, 70 (11): 1816–24.

Brown, S.J., Yelland, J.S., Sutherland, G.A., Baghurst, P.A. and Robinson, J.S. (2011) 'Stressful life events, social health issues and low birthweight in an Australian population-based birth cohort: challenges and opportunities in antenatal care', *BMC Public Health*, 11: 196.

Bryant, A.L., Schulenberg, J.E., O'Malley, P.M., Bachman J.G. and Johnston, L.D. (2003) 'How academic achievement, attitudes and behaviors relate to the course of substance use during adolescence: a 6-year, multiwave national longitudinal study', *Journal of Research on Adolescence*, 13 (3): 361–97.

Burdorf, A. (2010) 'Is early retirement good for your health?', *British Medical Journal*, 341: c6089. Doi: 10.1136/bmj.c6089.

Burns, R.A., Anstey, K.J. and Windsor, T.D. (2010) 'Subjective well-being mediates the effects of resilience and mastery on depression and anxiety in a large community sample of young and middle-aged adults', *Australian and New Zealand Journal of Psychiatry*, 45 (3): 240–8.

Burt, A., Maconochie, N., Doyle, P. and Roman, E. (2004) 'Learning difficulties in children born to male UK nuclear industry employees: analysis from the nuclear industry family study', *Occupational and Environmental Medicine*, 61 (9): 786–9.

Bury, M. (2000) 'Health, ageing and the lifecourse', in S.J. Williams, J. Gabe and M. Calnan (eds), *Health Medicine and Society: Key Theories, Future Agendas*. London: Routledge.

Busse, R., Blümel, M., Scheller-Kreinsen, D. and Zentner, A. (2010) *Tackling Chronic Disease in Europe*. Copenhagen: World Health Organization, on behalf of the European Observatory on Health Systems and Policies.

Cable, N., Bartley, M., McMunn, A. and Kelly, Y. (2010) 'Gender differences in the effect of breastfeeding on adult psychological well-being', *International Journal of Behavioural Medicine*, 17: 319.

Calafat, A., Blay, N.T., Hughes, K., Bellis, M., Juan, M., Duch, M. and Kokkevi, A. (2011) 'Nightlife young risk behaviours in Mediterranean versus other European cities: are stereotypes true?', *European Journal of Public Health*, 21 (3): 311–15.

Campbell, D. (2010) 'Cigarettes "to be sold in plain brown packs"', *Guardian*, 20 November, p. 11.

Campbell, F., Johnson, M., Messina, J., Guillaume, L. and Goyder, E. (2011) 'Behavioural interventions for weight management in pregnancy: a systematic review of quantitative and qualitative data', *BMC Public Health*, 11: 491.

Cancer Research UK (2011) *CancerStats: Incidence 2008, UK*. London: Cancer Research UK.

Cancer Research UK (2012) *Smoking: Statistics*, available at: http://info.cancerresearchuk. org/cancerstats/types/lung/smoking/#age

Carlson, D.L. (2011) 'Explaining the curvilinear relationship between age at first birth and depression among women', *Social Science and Medicine*, 72 (4): 494–503.

Case, A., Fertig, A. and Paxson, C. (2005) 'The lasting impact of childhood health and circumstance', *Journal of Health Economics*, 24 (2): 365–89.

Cattan, M., Kime, N. and Bagnal, A.-M. (2011) 'The use of telephone befriending in low-level support for socially isolated older people: an evaluation', *Health and Social Care in the Community*, 19 (2): 198–206.

Centre for Maternal and Child Enquiries (CMACE) (2007a) *Confidential Enquiry into Maternal and Child Health*. London: CMACE.

Centre for Maternal and Child Enquiries (CMACE) (2007b) *Diabetes in Pregnancy: Are we Providing the Best Care? Findings of a National Enquiry: England, Wales and Northern Ireland*. London: CMACE.

Centre for Maternal and Child Enquiries (CMACE) (2010) *Maternal Obesity in the UK: Findings for a National Project*. London: CMACE.

Chatzitheochari, S. and Arber, S. (2011) 'Identifying the third agers: an analysis of British retirees' leisure pursuits', *Sociological Research Online*, 16 (4): 3, available at: www. socresonline.org.uk/16/4/3.html10.5153/sro.2451

Chen, H., Cohen, P., Kasen, S., Johnson, J.G., Berenson, K. and Gordon, K. (2006) 'Impact of adolescent mental disorders and physical illnesses on quality of life 17 years later', *Archives of Pediatrics and Adolescent Medicine*, 160 (1): 93–9.

Claassen, L., Henneman, L., Janssens, A.C.J.W., Wijdenes-Pijl, M., Qureshi, N., Walter, F.M., Yoon, P.W. and Timmermans, D.R.M. (2010) 'Using family history information to promote healthy lifestyles and prevent diseases: a discussion of the evidence', *BMC Public Health*, 10: 24.

Clapham, D., Buckley, K., Mackie, P., Orford, S. and Stafford, I. (2010) *Young People and Housing in 2020: Identifying Key Drivers for Change*. York: Joseph Rowntree Foundation.

Cohen, G. (ed.) (1987) *Social Change and Life Course*. London: Tavistock Publications.

Coleman, J. (2007a) 'Emotional health and well-being', in J. Coleman, L. Hendry and M. Kloep (eds), *Adolescence and Health*. Chichester: John Wiley and Sons Ltd.

Coleman, J. (2007b) 'Sexual health', in J. Coleman, L. Hendry and M. Kloep (eds), *Adolescence and Health*. Chichester: John Wiley and Sons Ltd.

Coleman, J., Hendry, L. and Kloep, M. (2007) 'Understanding adolescent health', in J. Coleman, L. Hendry and M. Kloep (eds), *Adolescence and Health*. Chichester: John Wiley and Sons Ltd.

Collins, R.L., Ellickson, P.L. and Klein, D.J. (2007) 'The role of substance use in young adult divorce', *Addiction*, 102 (5): 786–94.

Connor, J., Gray, A. and Kypri, K. (2010) 'Drinking history, current drinking and problematic sexual experiences among university students', *Australian and New Zealand Journal of Public Health*, 34 (5): 487–94.

Crawshaw, M.A. and Sloper, P. (2010) '"Swimming against the tide": the influence of fertility matters on the transition to adulthood or survivorship following adolescent cancer', *European Journal of Cancer Care*, 19 (5): 610–20.

Crow, S.J. (2010) 'Eating disorders in young adults', in J.E. Grant and M.A. Potenza (eds), *Young Adult Mental Health*. New York: Oxford University Press.

Crowley, B.J., Hayslip, Jr, B. and Hobdy, J. (2003) 'Psychological hardiness and adjustment to life events in adulthood', *Journal of Adult Development*, 10 (4): 237–48.

Crump, C., Winkleby, M.A., Sundquist, K. and Sundquist, J. (2011a) 'Risk of asthma in young adults who were born preterm: a Swedish national cohort study', *Pediatrics*, 127 (4): 913–20.

Crump, C., Winkleby, M.A., Sundquist, K. and Sundquist, J. (2011b) 'Risk of hypertension among young adults who were born preterm: a Swedish national study of 636,000 births', *Pediatrics*, 173 (7): 797–803.

Darlington, R., Margo, J., Sternberg, S. and Karol Burks, B. (2011) *Through the Looking Glass*. London: Demos.

Dave, D.M. and Kelly, I.R. (2012) 'How does the business cycle affect eating habits?', *Social Science and Medicine*, 74 (2): 254–62.

Davey Smith, G. and Ebrahim, S. (2002) 'A life course approach to chronic disease epidemiology: conceptual models, empirical challenges and interdisciplinary perspectives', *International Journal of Epidemiology*, 32 (2): 285–93.

Davey Smith, G. and Lynch, D. (2005) 'Life course approaches to socioeconomic differential in health', in D. Kuh and Y. Ben-Shlomo (eds), *A Life Course Approach to Chronic Disease Epidemiology*, 2nd edn. Oxford: Oxford University Press).

Davey Smith, G., Gunnell, D. and Ben-Shlomo, Y. (2000) 'Life-course approaches to socio-economic differentials in cause specific adult mortality', in D. Leon and G. Walt (eds), *Poverty, Inequality and Health: An International Perspective*. Oxford: Oxford University Press.

Davidson, K. and Meadows, R. (2010) 'Older men's health: the role of marital status and masculinities', in B. Gough and S. Roberston (eds), *Men, Masculinities and Health: Critical Perspectives*. Basingstoke: Palgrave Macmillan.

Davies, K., Collerton, J.C., Jagger, C., Bond, J., Barker, S.A.H., Edwards, J., Hughes, J., Hunt, J.M. and Robinson, L. (2010) 'Engaging the oldest old in research: lessons from the Newcastle 85+ study', *BMC Geriatrics*, 10: 64.

Davis, E.P. and Sandman, C.A. (2006) 'Prenatal exposure to stress and stress hormones influences child development', *Infants and Young Children*, 19 (3): 246–59.

Davison, T.E., McCabe, M.P., Mellor, D., Ski, C., George, K. and Moore, K.A. (2007) 'The prevalence and recognition of major depression among low-level aged care residents with and without cognitive impairment', *Ageing and Mental Health*, 11 (1): 82–8.

de Ree, J. and Alessie, R. (2011) 'Life satisfaction and age: dealing with underidentifcation in age-period-cohort models', *Social Science and Medicine*, 73 (1): 177–82.

Debette, S. (2009) 'Parental dementia linked with compromised midlife memory in offspring', *American Academy of Neurology 61st Annual Meeting*, available at: www.medscape.com/viewarticle/588428

Degnen, C. (2007) 'Minding the gap: the construction of old age and oldness amongst peers', *Journal of Aging Studies*, 21 (1): 69–80.

Delisle, T.T., Werch, C.E., Wong, A.H., Bian, H. and Weiler, R. (2010) 'Relationship between frequency and intensity of physical activity and health behaviors of adolescents', *Journal of School Health*, 80 (3): 134–40.

Department for Work and Pensions (DWP) (2005) *Opportunity Age*. London: The Stationery Office.

Department for Work and Pensions (DWP) (2009) *Opportunity Age Indicators: 2008 Update*. London: DWP, Older People and Ageing Society Division.

Department of Health (2006) *The Health of Minority Ethnic Groups*. London: The Stationery Office.

Department of Health (2007) *The Pregnancy Book 2007*. London: Her Majesty's Stationery Office.

Department of Health (2008) *End of Life Care Strategy: Promoting High Quality Care for All Adults at the End of Life*. London: The Stationery Office.

Department of Health (2009a) *National Child Measurement Programme*. London: The Stationery Office.

Department of Health (2009b) *New Horizons: A Shared Vision for Mental Health*. London: Department of Health.

Department of Health (2009c) *The Pregnancy Book 2009*. London: The Stationery Office.

Department of Health (2010a) *A Vision for Adult Social Care: Capable Communities and Active Citizens*. London: Department of Health, available at: www.dh.gov.uk/publications

Department of Health (2010b) *Healthy Lives, Healthy People: Our Strategy for Public Health in England*. London: The Stationery Office.

Department of Health (2011a) *Health and Social Care Bill*. London: The Stationery Office.

Department of Health (2011b) *Mortality Monitoring Bulletin: Infant Mortality, Inequalities: Update to Include Data for 2010*. London: The Stationery Office.

Department of Health (2011c) *No Health without Mental Health*. London: The Stationery Office.

Desai, A. (2010) 'Governments confront drunken violence', *Bulletin of the World Health Organization*, 88 (9): 644–5.

Desai, S. (2000) 'Maternal education and child health: a feminist dilemma', *Feminist Studies*, 26 (2): 425–46.

Diener, E., Oishi, S. and. Lucas, R.E. (2003) 'Personality, culture, and subjective well-being: emotional and cognitive evaluations of life', *Annual Review of Psychology*, 54: 403–25.

Dike van de Mheen, H., Stronks, K. and Mackenbach, J.P. (1998) 'A lifecourse perspective on socio-economic inequalities in health: the influence of childhood socio-economic conditions and selection processes', *Sociology of Health and Illness*, 20 (5): 754–77.

DiPietro, J.A., Novak, M.F., Costigan, K.A., Atella, L.D. and Reusing, S.P. (2006) 'Maternal psychological distress during pregnancy in relation to child development at age 2', *Child Development*, 77 (3): 573–87.

Donath, C., Gräßel, E., Baierm, D., Pfeiffer, C., Karagülle, D., Bleich, S. and Hillemacher, T. (2011) 'Alcohol consumption and binge drinking in adolescents: comparison of different migration backgrounds and rural vs. urban residence – a representative study', *BMC Public Health*, 11: 84.

D'Onise, K., Lynch, J.W., McDermott, R.A. and Esterman, A. (2011) 'The beneficial effects of preschool attendance on adult cardiovascular disease risk', *Australian and New Zealand Journal of Public Health*, 35 (3): 278–83, doi: 10.1111/j.1753-6405.2010.00661.x.

dos Santos Silva, I. and de Stavola, B. (2002) 'Breast cancer aetiology: where do we go from here?', in D. Kuh and R. Hardy (eds), *A Life Course Approach to Women's Health*. Oxford: Oxford University Press.

Doyle, Y.G., McKee, M. and Sherriff, M. (2010) 'A model of successful ageing in British populations', *European Journal of Public Health*, 22 (1): 71–6.

Drenowatz, C., Eisenmann, J.C., Pfeiffer, K.A., Welk, G., Heelan, K., Gentile, D. and Walsh, D. (2010) 'Influence of socio-economic status on habitual physical activity and sedentary behavior in 8- to 11-year old children', *BMC Public Health*, 10: 214.

Dyson, L., McCormick, F. and Renfrew, M.J. (2007) 'Interventions for promoting the initiation of breastfeeding', *Cochrane Database of Systematic Reviews* 2005, (2), CD001688.

Eadie, D., MacAskill, S., Brooks, O., Heim, D., Forsyth, A. and Punc, S. (2010) *Pre-teens Learning about Alcohol: Drinking and Family Contexts*. York: Joseph Rowntree Foundation.

Eckersley, R. (2009) 'Population measures of subjective wellbeing: how useful are they?', *Social Indicators Research*, 94 (1): 1–12.

Ecob, R., Russ, S. and Davis, A. (2011) 'BMI over the life course and hearing ability at age 45 years: a population-based cohort study', *Longitudinal and Life Course Studies*, 2 (3): 242–59.

Economic and Social Research Council (2011) *Understanding Society: Early Findings from the First Wave of the UK's Household Longitudinal Study*. Swindon: Economic and Social Research Council.

Eilertsen, M.B., Rannestad, T., Rannestad, M.S. and Vik, T. (2011) 'Psychosocial health in children and adolescents surviving cancer', *Scandinavian Journal of Caring Sciences*, 25 (4): 725–34.

Eisenhower, A.S., Baker, B.L. and Blacher, J. (2009) 'Children's delayed development and behavior problems: impact on mothers' perceived physical health across early childhood', *Social Science and Medicine*, 68 (1): 89–99.

Eldh, A.C. and Carlsson, E. (2011) 'Seeking a balance between employment and the care of an ageing parent', *Scandinavian Journal of Caring Sciences*, 25 (2): 285–93.

Ely, G.E. and Dulmus, C.N. (2010) 'Disparities in access to reproductive health options for female adolescents', *Social Work in Public Health*, 25 (3): 341–51.

Emslie, C. and Hunt, K. (2009) '"Live to work" or "Work to live"? A qualitative study of gender and work–life balance among men and women in mid-life', *Gender, Work and Organization*, 16 (1): 151–72.

Emslie, C., Hunt, K. and Lyons, A. (2011) 'Older and wiser? Men's and women's accounts of drinking in early mid-life', *Sociology of Health and Illness*, 34: 481–96.

Entringer, S., Buss, C. and Wadhwa, P.D. (2010) 'Prenatal stress and developmental programming of human health and disease risk: concepts and integration of empirical findings', *Current Opinion in Endocrinology, Diabetes and Obesity*, 17 (6): 507–16.

Entringer, S., Wüst, S., Kumsta, R., Layes, I.M., Nelson, E.L., Hellhammer, D.H. and Wadhwa, P.D. (2008) 'Prenatal psychosocial stress exposure is associated with insulin resistance in young adults', *American Journal of Obstetrics and Gynaecology*, 199 (5): 498–505.

Eschmann, S., Zimprich, D., Metzke, C.W. and Steinhausen, H.-C. (2011) 'A developmental trajectory model of problematic substance use and psychosocial correlates from late adolescence to young adulthood', *Journal of Substance Use*, 16 (4): 295–312.

EuroHealthNet (2011) *Making the Link: Pensions and Health Equity*. Brussels: Equity Channel Publications.

EuroHealthNet (2012) *Healthy Ageing: The Importance of Technology*. Brussels: Equity Channel Publications.

European Social Survey (2011) *European Social Survey: Monitoring Attitude Change*. London: City University.

Fagerström, L. (2010) 'Positive life orientation: an inner health resource among older people', *Scandinavian Journal of Caring Sciences*, 24 (2): 349–56.

Faulkner, S. (2007) 'Eating disorders, dieting and body image', in J. Coleman, L. Hendry and M. Kloep (eds), *Adolescence and Health*. Chichester: John Wiley and Sons Ltd.

Fergusson, D.M. and Boden, J.M. (2008) 'Cannabis use and later life outcomes', *Addiction*, 103 (6): 969–76.

Ferri, C.P., Prince, M., Brayne, C., Brodaty, H., Fratiglioni, L., Ganguli, M., Hall, K., Hasegawa, K., Hendrie, H., Huang, Y., Jorm, A., Mathers, C., Menezes, P.R., Rimmer, E. and Scazufca, M. (2006) 'One hundred years on: global prevalence of dementia', *The Lancet*, 366 (9503): 2112–17.

Field, D. and Taylor, S. (eds) (2007) *Sociological Perspectives on Health, Illness and Health Care*, 4th edn. Oxford: Blackwell Science.

Field, F. (2010) *The Foundation Years: Preventing Poor Children Becoming Poor Adults*. London: Her Majesty's Stationery Office.

Finch, N. and Searle, B. (2005) 'Children's lifestyles', in J. Bradshaw and E. Mayhew (eds), *The Well-Being of Children in the UK*, 2nd edn. London: Save the Children Fund.

Fincham, F.D. and Beach, S.R.H. (2010) 'Marriage in the new millennium: a decade in review', *Journal of Marriage and Family*, 72 (3): 630–49.

Fisher, A., Saxton, J., Hill, C., Webber, L., Purslow, L. and Wardle, J. (2010) 'Psychosocial correlates of objectively measured physical activity in children', *European Journal of Public Health*, 21 (2): 145–50.

Fisher, A.J. and Gerein, N. (2008) 'Adolescents', in H.K. Hegginhoggan (ed.), *Encyclopaedia of Public Health*. San Diego, CA: Elsevier.

Foley, G., Alston, R., Geraci, M., Brabin, L., Kitchener, H. and Birch, J. (2011) 'Increasing rates of cervical cancer in young women in England: an analysis of national data 1982–2006', *British Journal of Cancer*, 105 (1): 177–84.

Fonseca, H., Matos, M.G., Guerra, A. and Gomes-Pedro, J. (2011) 'How much does overweight impact the adolescent developmental process?', *Child: Care, Health and Development*, 37 (1): 135–42.

Foot, C. and Harrison, T. (2011) *How to Improve Cancer Survival: Explaining England's Relatively Poor Rates*. London: The King's Fund.

Foresight Report (2007) *Trends and Drivers of Obesity: A Literature Review for the Foresight Project on Obesity*. London: Government Office for Science.

Fox, N., Ward, K. and O'Rourke, A. (2005) 'Pro-anorexia, weight-loss drugs and the internet: an "anti-recovery" explanatory model of anorexia', *Sociology of Health and Illness*, 27 (7): 944–71.

Freedman, V.A., Stafford, F., Schwarz, N., Conrad, F. and Cornman, J.C. (2012) 'Disability, participation, and subjective wellbeing among older couples', *Social Science and Medicine*, 74 (4): 588–96.

Freunscht, I. and Feldmann, R. (2011) 'Young adults with fetal alcohol syndrome (FAS): social, emotional and occupational development', *Klinische Padiatrie*, 223 (1): 33–7.

Friedli, L. (2009) *Mental Health, Resilience and Inequalities*. Copenhagen: World Health Organization.

Friedman, H.S., Tucker, J.S., Tomlinson-Keasey, C., Schwartz, J.E., Wingard, D.L. and Criqui, M.H. (1993) 'Does childhood personality predict longevity?', *Journal of Personality and Social Psychology*, 65: 176–85.

Fuller, E. and Sanchez, M. (eds) (2010) *Smoking, Drinking and Drug Abuse among Young People in England in 2009*. London: NHS Information Centre for Health and Social Care.

Gammell, C. (2009) 'Middle-aged women suffering most from mental health problems', *Telegraph*, 27 January, p. 7.

Garber, J., Ciesla, J.A., McCauley, E., Diamond, G. and Schloredt, K.A. (2011) 'Remission of depression in parents: links to healthy functioning in their children', *Child Development*, 82 (1): 226–42.

Garthus-Niegel, S., Knut A., Hagtvet, K.A. and Vollrath, M.E. (2010) 'A prospective study of weight development and behavior problems in toddlers: the Norwegian Mother and Child Cohort Study', *BMC Public Health*, 10: 626.

Gatrell, C. (2008) *Embodying Women's Work*. Maidenhead: McGraw-Hill.

Gaudineau, A., Ehlinger, V., Vayssiere, C., Jouret, B., Arnau, C. and Godeau, E. (2010) 'Factors associated with early menarche: results from the French Health Behaviour in School-Aged Children (HBSC) study', *BMC Public Health*, 10: 175.

Geijer, R.M.M., Sachs, A.P.E., Verheij, T.J.M., Salomé, P.L., Lammers, J.-W.J. and Hoes, A.W. (2006) 'Incidence and determinants of moderate COPD (GOLD II) in male smokers aged 40–65 years: 5-year follow-up', *British Journal of General Practice*, 56 (530): 656–61.

Gerhardt, S. (2006) *Why Love Matters: How Affection Shapes a Baby's Brain*. London: Routledge.

Gerward, S., Tydén, P., Engström, G. and Hedblad, B. (2010) 'Marital status and occupation in relation to short-term case fatality after a first coronary event: a population-based cohort', *BMC Public Health*, 10: 235.

Gibb, S.J., Fergusson, D.M. and Horwood, L.J. (2010) 'Burden of psychiatric disorder in young adulthood and life outcomes at age 30', *British Journal of Psychiatry*, 197 (2): 122–7.

Gibbs, I., Sinclair, I. and Stein, M. (2005). 'Children and young people in and leaving care', in J. Bradshaw and E. Mayhew (eds), *The Well-Being of Children in the UK*, 2nd edn. London: Save the Children Fund.

Giles, L.C., Glonek, G.F.V., Moore, V.M., Davies, M.J. and Luszcz, M.A. (2010) 'Lower age at menarche affects survival in older Australian women: results from the Australian Longitudinal Study of Ageing', *BMC Public Health*, 10: 341.

Gill, T. (2007) *No Fear: Growing up in a Risk Averse Society*. London: Calouste Gulbenkian Foundation.

Gillman, M. (2005) 'A life course approach to obesity', in D. Kuh and Y. Ben-Shlomo (eds), *A Life Course Approach to Chronic Disease Epidemiology*, 2nd edn. Oxford: Oxford University Press.

Giskes, K., Turrell, G., Bentley, R. and Kavanagh. A. (2011) 'Individual and household-level socioeconomic position is associated with harmful alcohol consumption behaviours among adults', *Australian and New Zealand Journal of Public Health*, 35 (3): 270–7.

Glaser, K., Evandrou, M. and Tomassini, C. (2006) 'Multiple role occupancy and social participation among midlife wives and husbands in the United Kingdom', *International Journal of Aging and Human Development*, 63 (1): 27–47.

Glendinning, C., Kloep, M. and Hendry, L.B. (2000) 'Parenting practices and well-being in youth: family life in rural Scotland and Sweden', in H. Ryan and J. Bull (eds), *Changing Families, Changing Communities: Researching Health and Well-Being among Children and Young People*. London: Health Development Agency.

Goodman, S.H. and Rous, M.H. (2010) *Perinatal Depression and Children: A Developmental*. Montreal: Centre of Excellence for Early Childhood Development.

Graham, H. (2002) 'Building an inter-disciplinary science of health inequalities: the example of life course research', *Social Science and Medicine*, 55 (11): 2005–16.

Graham, H. (2007) *Unequal Lives: Health and Socioeconomic Inequalities*. Maidenhead: Open University Press.

Graham, H. (ed.) (2009) *Understanding Health Inequalities*, 2nd edn. Maidenhead: McGraw-Hill.

Graham, H. and Power, C. (2004) 'Childhood disadvantage and health inequalities: a framework for policy based on life course research', *Child: Care, Health and Development*, 30 (6): 671–8.

Graham, S. (2010) *Home Truths, 2010: Why Investment in Affordable Housing Matters*. London: National Housing Federation.

Gralinski-Bakker, J.H., Hauser, S., Billings, R., Allen, J., Lyons, P. and Melton, G. (2005) *Transitioning to Adulthood for Young Adults with Mental Health Issues* (Network on Transitions to Adulthood Policy Brief). Philadelphia, PA: MacArthur Foundation Research Network on Transitions to Adulthood and Public Policy, University of Pennsylvania.

Grant, J.E. and Potenza, M.A. (eds) (2010) *Young Adult Mental Health*. New York: Oxford University Press.

Gray, C.M., Hunt, K., Lorimer, K., Anderson, A.S., Benzeval, M. and Wyke, S. (2011) 'Words matter: a qualitative investigation of which weight status terms are acceptable and motivate weight loss when used by health professionals', *BMC Public Health*, 11: 513.

Green, L. (2010) *Understanding the Life Course: Sociological and Psychological Perspectives*. Cambridge: Polity Press.

Grinyer, A. (2007) *Young People Living with Cancer*. Maidenhead: McGraw-Hill.

Grinyer, A. (2009) *Life after Cancer in Adolescence and Young Adulthood: The Experience of Survivorship*. Abingdon: Routledge.

Gruenewald, T.L., Karlamangla, A.S., Hu, P., Stein-Merkin, S., Crandall, C., Koretz, B. and Seeman, T.E. (2012) 'History of socioeconomic disadvantage and allostatic load in later life', *Social Science and Medicine*, 74 (11): 75–83.

Grundy, E.M.D. and Tomassini, C. (2010) 'Marital history, health and mortality among older men and women in England and Wales', *BMC Public Health*, 10: 554.

Gunderson, E.P., Matias, S.L., Hurston, S.R., Dewey, K.G., Ferrara, A., Quesenberry, C.P., Lo, J.C., Sternfeld, B. and Selby, J.V. (2011) 'Study of women, infant feeding, and Type 2 diabetes mellitus after GDM pregnancy (SWIFT), a prospective cohort study: methodology and design', *BMC Public Health*, 11: 952.

Gunnarsson, E. (2009) '"I think I have had a good life": the everyday lives of older women and men from a life course perspective', *Ageing and Society*, 29 (1): 33–48.

Guo, H.J., McGee, R., Reeder, T. and Gray, A. (2010) 'Smoking behaviours and contextual influences on adolescent nicotine dependence', *Australian and New Zealand Journal of Public Health*, 34 (5): 502–7.

Hall, B. and Place, M. (2010) 'Cutting to cope: a modern adolescent phenomenon', *Child: Care, Health and Development*, 36 (5): 623–9.

Hallfors, D.D., Waller, M.W., Ford, C.A., Halpern, C.T., Brodish, P.H. and Iritani, B. (2004) 'Adolescent depression and suicide risk: association with sex and drug behavior', *American Journal of Preventive Medicine*, 27 (3): 224–31.

Hallgren, M.A., Högberg, P. and Andréasson, S. (2010) 'Alcohol consumption and harm among elderly Europeans: falling between the cracks', *European Journal of Public Health*, 20 (6): 616–17.

Halpern, C.T. (2010) 'Reframing research on adolescent sexuality: healthy sexual development as part of the life course', *Perspectives on Sexual and Reproductive Health*, 42 (1): 6–7.

Hanratty, B., Drever, F., Jacoby, A. and Whitehead, M. (2007) 'Retirement age caregivers and deprivation of area of residence in England and Wales', *European Journal of Ageing*, 4 (1): 35–43.

Hardy, R. and Kuh, D. (2002) 'Menopause and gynaecological disorders: a life course perspective', in D. Kuh and R. Hardy (eds), *A Life Course Approach to Women's Health*. Oxford: Oxford University Press.

Hareven, T.K. (1995) 'Changing images of aging and the social construction of the life course', in M. Featherstone and A. Wernick (eds), *Images of Aging: Cultural Representations of Later Life*. London: Routledge.

Harris, J.R. (1998) *The Nurture Assumption: Why Children Turn out the Way They Do*. New York: Free Press.

Harris, P. (2010) 'Health concerns over boom in anti-age therapy', *Observer*, 5 September, p. 12.

Harrison, F., Jones, A.P., van Sluijs, E.M.F., Cassidy, A., Bentham, G. and Griffin, S.J. (2011a) 'Environmental correlates of adiposity in 9–10 year old children: considering home and school neighbourhoods and routes to school', *Social Science and Medicine*, 72 (9): 1411–19.

Harrison, K., Bost, K.K., McBride, B.A., Donovan, S.M., Grigsby-Toussaint, D.S., Kim, J., Liechty, J.M., Wiley, A., Teran-Garcia, M. and Costa Jacobsohn, G. (2011b) 'Toward a developmental conceptualization of contributors to overweight and obesity in childhood: the six-Cs model', *Child Development Perspectives*, 5 (1): 50–8.

Hart, C.L., Davey Smith, G., Gruer, L. and Watt, G.C.M. (2010) 'The combined effect of smoking tobacco and drinking alcohol on cause-specific mortality: a 30-year cohort study', *BMC Public Health*, 10: 789.

Hart, C.N., Raynor, H.A., Jelalian, E. and Drotar, D. (2010) 'The association of maternal food intake and infants' and toddlers' food intake', *Child: Care, Health and Development*, 36 (3): 396–403.

Harvey, K.J., Brown, B., Crawford, P., Macfarlane, A. and McPherson, A. (2007) '"Am I normal?" Teenagers, sexual health and the Internet', *Social Science and Medicine*, 65: 771–81.

Hauge, S. and Kirkevold, M. (2012) 'Variations in older persons' descriptions of the burden of loneliness', *Scandinavian Journal of Caring Sciences*, 26 (3): 553–60.

Health Protection Agency (2009) *National Chlamydia Screening Programme*, 3rd edn. London: Health Protection Agency.

Health Protection Agency (2011) *HIV in the United Kingdom: 2011 Report*. London: Health Protection Agency.

Heffner, K.L., Waring, M.E., Roberts, M.B., Eaton, C.B. and Gramling, R. (2011) 'Social isolation, C-reactive protein, and coronary heart disease mortality among community-dwelling adults', *Social Science and Medicine*, 72 (9): 1482–8.

Heikkilä, K., Sacker, A., Kelly, Y., Renfrew, M.J. and Quigley, M.A. (2011) 'Breast feeding and child behaviour in the Millennium Cohort Study', *Archives of Disease in Childhood*, 96 (7): 635–42.

Helm, T. (2010) 'Don't ruin the health of our children's schools plead after cuts to sport cash', *Observer*, 21 November, p. 8.

Helms, P.J. (2007) 'Being different: adolescents, chronic illness and disability', in J. Coleman, L. Hendry and M. Kloep (eds), *Adolescence and Health*. Chichester: John Wiley and Sons Ltd.

Hendrie, G.A., Covene, J. and Cox, D.N. (2011) 'Factor analysis shows association between family activity environment and children's health behaviour', *Australian and New Zealand Journal of Public Health*, 356 (6): 524–9.

Her Majesty's Treasury (2004) *Spending Review: Public Service Agreements 2005–2008*. London: Her Majesty's Stationery Office.

Hester, R.K., Squires, D.D. and Delaney, H.D. (2005) 'The drinker's check-up: 12-month outcomes of a controlled clinical trial of a stand-alone software program for problem drinkers', *Journal of Substance Abuse Treatment*, 28 (2): 159–69.

Hillsdon, M., Foster, C., Naidoo, B. and Crombie, H. (2005) *The Effectiveness of Public Health Interventions for Increasing Physical Activity among Adults: A Review of Reviews, Evidence Briefing*. London: National Institute for Health and Clinical Excellence.

Hockey, J. and James, A. (2003) *Social Identities across the Life Course*. Basingstoke: Palgrave Macmillan.

Hoeck, S., François, G., Geerts, J., Van der Heyden, J., Vandewoude, M. and Van Hal, G. (2011) 'Health-care and home-care utilization among frail elderly persons in Belgium', *European Journal of Public Health*, doi: 10.1093/eurpub/ckr133.

Hogan, A.H., Howell-Jones, R.S., Pottinger, E., Wallace, L.M. and McNulty, C.A.M. (2010) '"...they should be offering it": a qualitative study to investigate young peoples' attitudes towards chlamydia screening in GP surgeries', *BMC Public Health*, 10: 616.

Holme, A., MacArthur, C. and Lancashire, R. (2010) 'The effects of breastfeeding on cognitive and neurological development of children at 9 years', *Child: Care, Health and Development*, 36 (4): 583–90.

Holstein, J.A. and Gubrium, J.F. (2000) *Constructing the Life Course*. New York: General Hall, Inc.

Holt, A. (2011) 'The terrorist in my home: teenagers' violence towards parents – constructions of parent experiences in public online message boards', *Child and Family Social Work*, 16 (4): 454–63.

Hooper, C. (2005) 'Child maltreatment', in J. Bradshaw and E. Mayhew (eds), *The Well-Being of Children in the UK*, 2nd edn. London: Save the Children Fund.

Hopkins Tanne, J. (2010) 'Babies born at night have higher risk of encephalopathy, Californian study shows', *British Medical Journal*, 341: c7036.

Hosking, J., Ameratunga, S., Morton, S. and Blank, D. (2011) 'A life course approach to injury prevention: a "lens and telescope" conceptual model', *BMC Public Health*, 11: 695.

Hughes, S.K., Hughes, K., Atkinson, A.M., Bellis, M.A. and Smallthwaite, L. (2011) 'Smoking behaviours, access to cigarettes and relationships with alcohol in 15- and 16-year-old schoolchildren', *European Journal of Public Health*, 21 (1): 8–14.

Humensky, J.L. (2010) 'Are adolescents with high socioeconomic status more likely to engage in alcohol and illicit drug use in early adulthood?', *Substance Abuse: Treatment, Prevention, and Policy*, 5: 19.

Hunt, K., Sweeting, H., Keoghan, M., and Platt, S. (2006) 'Sex, gender role orientation, gender role attitudes and suicidal thoughts in three generations: a general population study', *Social Psychiatry and Psychiatric Epidemiology*, 41 (8): 641–7.

Hunt, S. (2005) *The Life Course: A Sociological Introduction*. Basingstoke: Palgrave Macmillan.

Jackson, S. and Scott, S. (2006) 'Childhood', in G. Payne (ed.), *Social Divisions*. Basingstoke: Macmillan.

Jago, R., Fox, K.R., Page, A.S., Brockman, R. and Thompson, J.L. (2010) 'Parent and child physical activity and sedentary time: do active parents foster active children?', *BMC Public Health*, 10: 194.

Järvinen, M. and Ravn, S. (2011) 'From recreational to regular drug use: qualitative interviews with young clubbers', *Sociology of Health and Illness*, 33 (4): 554–69.

Johnson, R.C., Schoeni, R.F. and Rogowski, J.A. (2012) 'Health disparities in mid-to-late life: the role of earlier life family and neighborhood socioeconomic conditions', *Social Science and Medicine*, 74 (4): 625–36.

Jonas, S., Bebbington, P., McManus, S., Meltzer, H., Jenkins, R., Kuipers, E., Cooper, C., King, M. and Brugha, T. (2011) 'Sexual abuse and psychiatric disorder in England: results from the 2007 adult psychiatric morbidity survey', *Psychological Medicine*, 41 (4): 709–19.

Joseph, K.S. and Kramer, M.S. (2005) 'Should we intervene to improve fetal and infant growth?', in D. Kuh. and Y. Ben-Shlomo (eds), *A Life Course Approach to Chronic Disease Epidemiology*, 2nd edn. Oxford: Oxford University Press.

Jotangia, D., Ogunbadejo, T. and Simmonds, N. (2010) 'Drug use', in E. Fuller and M. Sanchez (eds), *Smoking, Drinking and Drug Abuse among Young People in England in 2009*. London: NHS Information Centre for Health and Social Care.

Joyce, K. and Loe, M. (2010) 'A sociological approach to ageing, technology and health', *Sociology of Health and Illness*, 32 (2): 171–80.

Kahneman, D., Krueger, A.B., Schkade, D., Schwarz, N. and Stone, A. (2004) 'Toward national well-being accounts', *American Economic Review*, 9: 429–34.

Katz, J., Holland, C., Peace, S. and Taylor, E. (2011) *A Better Life: What Older People with High Support Needs Value*. York: Joseph Rowntree Foundation.

Keller, S.K. and Schulz, P.J. (2010) 'Distorted food pyramid in kids' programmes: a content analysis of television advertising watched in Switzerland', *European Journal of Public Health*, 21 (3): 300–5.

Kelly, Y.J. and Watt, R.G. (2005) 'Breastfeeding initiation and exclusive duration at 6 months by social class: results from the Millennium Cohort Study', *Public Health Nutrition*, 8 (4): 417–21.

Kerr, D.C.R. and Capaldi, D. (2011) 'Young men's intimate partner violence and relationship functioning: long-term outcomes associated with suicide attempt and aggression in adolescence', *Psychological Medicine*, 41 (4): 759–69.

Kidger, J., Donovan, J.L., Biddle, L., Campbell, R. and Gunnell, D. (2009) 'Supporting adolescent emotional health in schools: a mixed methods study of student and staff views in England', *BMC Public Health*, 9: 403.

Kim, M.J., Catalano, R.F., Haggerty, K.P. and Abbott, R.D. (2011) 'Bullying at elementary school and problem behaviour in young adulthood: a study of bullying, violence and substance use from age 11 to age 21', *Criminal Behaviour and Mental Health*, 21 (2): 136–44.

Kimbro, R.T. (2008) 'Together forever? Romantic relationship characteristics and prenatal health behaviors', *Journal of Marriage and Family*, 70 (3): 745–57.

King, A.C., Parkinson, K., Adamson, A.J., Murray, L., Besson, H., Reilly, J.J. and Basterfield, L. (2010) 'Correlates of objectively measured physical activity and sedentary behaviour in English children', *European Journal of Public Health*, 21 (4): 424–31.

Klijs, B., Mackenbach, J.P. and Kunst, A.E. (2011) 'Obesity, smoking, alcohol consumption and years lived with disability: a Sullivan life table approach', *BMC Public Health*, 11: 378.

Knapp, M., McDaid, D. and Parsonage M. (eds) (2011) *Mental Health Promotion and Mental Illness Prevention: The Economic Case*. London: Department of Health.

Koshy, P., Mackenzie, M., Tappin, D. and Bauld, L. (2010) 'Smoking cessation during pregnancy: the influence of partners, family and friends on quitters and non-quitters', *Health and Social Care in the Community*, 18 (5) 500–10.

Kramer, M., Cooper, H.L., Drews-Botsch, C.D., Waller, L.A. and Hogue, C.R. (2010) 'Metropolitan isolation segregation and Black–White disparities in very preterm birth: a test of mediating pathways and variance explained', *Social Science and Medicine*, 71: 2108–16.

Kravdal, H. and Syse, A. (2011) 'Changes over time in the effect of marital status on cancer survival', *BMC Public Health*, 11: 804.

Kubzansky, L.D., Martin, L.T. and Buka, S.L. (2009) 'Early manifestations of personality and adult health: a life course perspective', *Health Psychology*, 28 (3): 364–72.

Kuh, D. and Ben-Shlomo, Y. (eds) (2005) *A Life Course Approach to Chronic Disease Epidemiology*, 2nd edn. Oxford: Oxford University Press.

Kuh, D. and Hardy, R. (eds) (2002) *A Life Course Approach to Women's Health*. Oxford: Oxford University Press.

Kuh, D. and Wadsworth, M. (1993) 'Physical health status at 36 years in a British national birth cohort', *Social Science and Medicine*, 37 (7): 905–16.

Kuh, D., Power, C., Blane, D. and Bartley, M. (2005) 'Socioeconomic pathways between childhood and adult health', in D. Kuh and Y. Ben-Shlomo (eds), *A Life Course Approach to Chronic Disease Epidemiology*, 2nd edn. Oxford: Oxford University Press.

Kuramoto, S.J., Stuart, E., Runeson, B., Lichtenstein, P., Langstrom, N. and Wilcox, H.C. (2010) 'Maternal versus paternal suicide and offspring risk of hospitalization for psychiatric disorders and suicide attempt', *Pediatrics*, 126 (5): 1026–32.

Kwansa, T. (2007) 'Adolescent risk taking in sexual behaviours', in J.L. Leishman and J. Moir (eds), *Pre-teen and Teenage Pregnancy: A Twenty-First-Century Reality*. Keswick: M&K Publishing Ltd.

Landau, R., Avital, M., Berger, A., Atzaba-Poria, N., Arbelle, S., Faroy, M. and Auerbach, J.G. (2010) 'Parenting of 7-month-old infants at familial risk for attention deficit/hyperactivity disorder', *Infant Mental Health Journal*, 31 (2): 141–58.

Landstedt, E., Asplund, K. and Gillander Gådin, K. (2009) 'Understanding adolescent mental health: the influence of social processes, doing gender and gendered power relations', *Sociology of Health and Illness*, 31 (7): 962–78.

Larkin, M. (2009) *Vulnerable Groups in Health and Social Care*. London: Sage.

Larkin, M. (2011a) *Social Aspects of Health, Illness and Healthcare*. Maidenhead: McGraw-Hill.

Larkin, M. (2011b) 'What about the carers?', in T.D. Heller and C.E. Lloyd (eds), *Long Term Conditions: Challenges in Health and Social Care Practice*. London: Sage.

Law, C. (2009) 'Life influences on children's futures', in H. Graham (ed.), *Understanding Health Inequalities*. Maidenhead: McGraw-Hill.

Lawlor, D.A., Benfield, L., Logue, J., Tilling, K., Howe, L.D., Fraser, A., Cherry, L., Watt, P., Ness, A.R., Davey Smith, G. and Sattar, N. (2010) 'Association between general and central adiposity in childhood, and change in these, with cardiovascular risk factors in adolescence: prospective cohort study', *British Medical Journal*, 341: c6224.

Leach, P. (2010) *The Essential First Year*. London: Dorling Kindersley Publishers Ltd.

Lee, E. (2010) 'Pathologising fatherhood: the case of male post-natal depression in Britain', in B. Gough and S. Roberston (eds), *Men, Masculinities and Health: Critical Perspectives*. Basingstoke: Palgrave Macmillan.

Legleye, S., Obradovic, I., Janssen, E., Spilka, S., Le Nézet, O. and Beck, F. (2009) 'Influence of cannabis use trajectories, grade repetition and family background on the school-dropout rate at the age of 17 years in France', *European Journal of Public Health*, 20 (2): 157–63.

Leishman, J.L. (2007) 'Pre-teen and teenage pregnancy', in J.L. Leishman and J. Moir (eds), *Pre-teen and Teenage Pregnancy: A Twenty-First-Century Reality*. Keswick: M&K Publishing Ltd.

Leishman, J.L. and Moir, J. (eds) (2007) *Pre-teen and Teenage Pregnancy: A Twenty-First-Century Reality*. Keswick: M&K Publishing Ltd.

Levinson, D.J. (1978) *The Seasons of a Man's Life*. New York: Ballantine.

Lindeberg, S.I., Rosvall, M., Choi, B.-K., Canivet, C., Isacsson, S.-O., Karasek, R. and Östergren, P.-O. (2011) 'Psychosocial working conditions and exhaustion in a working population sample of Swedish middle-aged men and women', *European Journal of Public Health*, 21 (2): 190–6.

Lindvall, K., Larsson, L., Weinehall, L. and Emmelin, M. (2010) 'Weight maintenance as a tight rope walk: a Grounded Theory study', *BMC Public Health*, 10: 51.

Littlefield, A.K. and Sher, K.J. (2010) 'Alcohol use disorders in young adulthood', in J.E. Grant and M.A. Potenza (eds), *Young Adult Mental Health*. New York: Oxford University Press.

Lloyd, C.E. and Skinner, T.C. (2009) 'Policy and practice for diabetes care', in E. Denny and S. Earle (eds), *The Sociology of Long-term Conditions and Nursing Practice*. Basingstoke: Palgrave Macmillan.

Loucks, E.B., Abrahamowicz, M., Xiao, Y. and Lynch, J.W. (2011) ' Associations of education with 30-year life course blood pressure trajectories: Framingham Offspring Study', *BMC Public Health*, 11: 139.

Lovasi, G.S., Quinn, J.W., Rauh, V.A., Perera, F.P., Andrews, H.F., Garfinkel, R., Hoepner, L., Whyatt, R. and Rundle, A. (2010) 'Chlorpyrifos exposure and urban residential environment characteristics as determinants of early childhood neurodevelopment', *American Journal of Public Health*, online 101 (1): 63–70.

Lowry, R., Kremer, J. and Trew, K. (2007) 'Young people: physical health, exercise and recreation', in J. Coleman, L. Hendry and M. Kloep (eds), *Adolescence and Health*. Chichester: John Wiley and Sons Ltd.

Lu, M.C., Kotelchuck, M., Hohan, V., Jones, L., Wright, K. and Halfon, N. (2010) 'Closing the Black–White gap in birth outcomes; a life-course approach', *Ethnicity and Disease*, 20 (1, Suppl. 2): S62–76.

Luo, Y., Hawkley, L.C., Waite, L.J. and Cacioppo, J.T. (2012) 'Loneliness, health, and mortality in old age: a national longitudinal study', *Social Science and Medicine*, 74 (6): 907–14.

Lynch, J.W. and Davey Smith, G. (2005) 'A life course approach to chronic disease epidemiology', *Annual Review of Public Health*, 26: 1–35.

Lynch, J.W., Kaplan, G. and Salonen, J.T. (1997) 'Why do poor people behave poorly? Variations in adult health behaviours and psychosocial characteristics by stages of the socio-economic life course', *Social Science and Medicine*, 44 (6): 809–19.

Lynch, J.W., Law, C., Brinkman, S., Chittleborough, C. and Sawyer, M. (2010) 'Inequalities in child healthy development: some challenges for effective implementation', *Social Science and Medicine*, 71 (7): 1244–8.

Macfarlane, A. and McPherson, A. (2007) 'Getting it right in health services for young people', in J. Coleman, L. Hendry and M. Kloep (eds), *Adolescence and Health*. Chichester: John Wiley and Sons Ltd.

Majer, I.M., Nusselder, W.J., Mackenbach, J.P. and Kunst, A.E. (2011) 'Socioeconomic inequalities in life and health expectancies around official retirement age in 10 Western-European countries', *Journal of Epidemiology and Community Health*, 65: 972–9.

Mandal, B., Ayyagari, P. and Gallo, W.T. (2011) 'Job loss and depression: the role of subjective expectations', *Social Science and Medicine*, 72 (8): 576–83.

Marmot, M. (2010) *Fair Society, Healthy Lives: A Strategic Review of Health Inequalities in England Post-2010 (Marmot Review)*. London: The Marmot Review.

Marmot Review Team (2011) *The Health Impacts of Cold Homes and Fuel Poverty*. London: The Marmot Review.

Marshall, N.L. and Tracy, A.J. (2009) 'After the baby: work–family conflict and working mothers' psychological health', *Family Relations*, 58 (4): 380–91.

Martin, L.G., Schoeni, R.F., Freedman, V.A. and Andreski, P. (2007) 'Feeling better? Trends in general health status', *Journals of Gerontology*, 62 (1): 11–21.

Martin, R.M., Ben-Shlomo, Y., Gunnell, D., Elwood, P., Yarnell, J.W. and Davey Smith, G. (2005) 'Breast feeding and cardiovascular disease risk factors, incidence, and mortality: the Caerphilly study', *Journal of Epidemiology and Community Health*, 59 (2): 121–9.

Martín-Matillas, M., Ortega, F.B., Ruiz, J.R., Martínez-Gómez, D., Marcos, A., Moliner-Urdiales, D., Polito, A., Pedrero-Chamizo, R., Béghin, L., Molnár, D., Kafatos, A., Moreno, L.A., De Bourdeaudhui, I. and Sjöström, M. (2010) 'Adolescents' physical activity levels and relatives' physical activity engagement and encouragement: the HELENA study', *European Journal of Public Health*, 21 (6): 705–12.

Mayhew, E., Finch, N., Beresford, B. and Keung, A. (2005) 'Children's time and space', in J. Bradshaw and E. Mayhew (eds), *The Well-Being of Children in the UK*, 2nd edn. London: Save the Children Fund.

Mayhew, L., Richardson, J. and and Rickayzen, B. (2009) 'A study into the detrimental effects of obesity on life expectancy in the UK', available at: www.actuaries.org.uk/research-and-resources/documents/study-detrimental-effects-obesity-life-expectancy-uk.

McCarron, P., Smith, G.D., Okasha, M. and McEwen, J. (2000) 'Blood pressure in young adulthood and mortality from cardiovascular disease', *The Lancet*, 355 (9213): 1430–1.

McCarthy, H. and Thomas, G. (2004) *Home Alone: Combating Isolation with Older Housebound People*. London: Demos.

McColl, K. (2010) 'Experts pool ideas on how to cut maternal mortality', *British Medical Journal*, 341: c5017.

McConkey, R., Truesdale-Kennedy, M., Chang, M.-Y., Jarrah, S. and Shukri, R. (2008) 'The impact on mothers of bringing up a child with intellectual disabilities: a cross-cultural study', *International Journal of Nursing Studies*, 45 (1): 65–74.

McCormick, J., Clifton, J., Sachrajda, A., Cherti, M. and McDowell, E. (2009) *Getting on: Well-Being in Later Life*. London: Institute for Public Policy Research.

McCrone, P., Dhanasiri, S., Patel, A., Knapp, M. and Lawton-Smith, S. (2008) *Paying the Price: The Cost of Mental Health Care in England to 2026*. London: The King's Fund.

McCrory, C. and Layte, R. (2011) 'The effect of breastfeeding on children's educational test scores at nine years of age: results of an Irish cohort study', *Social Science and Medicine*, 72 (9): 1515–21.

McGauran, A. (2010) 'Over 55s in US are less healthy than their English peers but live longer', *British Medical Journal*, 341: c6311, doi: 10.1136/bmj.c6311.

McGorry, P.D., Purcell, R., Goldstone, S. and Amminger G.P. (2011) 'Age of onset and timing of treatment for mental and substance use disorders: implications for preventive intervention strategies and models of care', *Current Opinion in Psychiatry*, 24 (4): 301–6.

McMahon, T. (2010) 'Developmental pathways to parenting', in J.E. Grant and M.N. Potenza (eds), *Young Adult Mental Health*. New York: Oxford University Press.

McVeigh, T. (2011) 'Breast feeding makes babies more intelligent, claim scientists', *Observer*, 13 March, p. 26.

McVicar, D. (2011) 'Estimates of peer effects in adolescent smoking across twenty-six European countries', *Social Science and Medicine*, 73 (8): 1186–93.

Meltzer, H., Doos, L., Vostanis, P., Ford, T. and Goodman, R. (2009) 'The mental health of children who witness domestic violence', *Child and Family Social Work*, 14 (4): 491–501.

Meltzer, H., Gatward, R., Corbin, T., et al. (2003) *Persistence, Onset, Risk Factors and Outcomes of Childhood Mental Disorders*. London: Office for National Statistics.

Mensah, F.K. and Kiernan, K.E. (2011) 'Maternal general health and children's cognitive development and behaviour in the early years: findings from the Millennium Cohort Study', *Child: Care, Health and Development*, 37 (10): 44–54.

Mertens, V.-C., Bosma, H., Groffen, D.A.I. and van Eijk, J.T.M. (2011) 'Good friends, high income or resilience? What matters most for elderly patients?', *European Journal of Public Health*, 22 (5): 666–71.

Milkie, M.A., Norris, D.R. and Bierman, A. (2011) 'The long arm of offspring: adult children's troubles as teenagers and elderly parents' mental health', *Research on Aging*, 33 (3): 327–55.

Miller, D. (2011) 'Associations between the home and school environments and child body mass index', *Social Science and Medicine*, 72 (5): 677–84.

Minet Kinge, J. and Morris, S. (2010) 'Socioeconomic variation in the impact of obesity on health-related quality of life', *Social Science and Medicine*, 71 (10): 677–84.

Mitchell, D.B. and Hauser-Cram, P. (2008) 'The well-being of mothers of adolescents with developmental disabilities in relation to medical care utilization and satisfaction with health care', *Research in Developmental Disabilities*, 29 (2): 97–112.

Morgen, C.S., Mortensen, L.H., Rasmussen, M., Andersen, A.M., Sørensen, T.I. and Due, P. (2010) 'Parental socioeconomic position and development of overweight in adolescence: longitudinal study of Danish adolescents', *BMC Public Health*, 10: 520.

Musacchio, N.S. and Forcier, M. (2008) 'Adolescent health', *International Encyclopaedia of Public Health*, 43 (2): 201–4.

Nabieva, T.N. (2007) 'Physical and neurological state of the newborn after the perinatal asphyxia', *Uspekhi Fiziologicheskikh Nauk*, 38 (4): 73–9.

Nabkasorn, C., Miyai, N., Sootmongkol, A., Junprasert, S., Yamamoto, H., Arita, M. and Miyashita, K. (2005) 'Effects of physical exercise on depression, neuroendocrine stress hormones and physiological fitness in adolescent females with depressive symptoms', *European Journal of Public Health*, 16 (2): 179–84.

Nagle, C., Skouteris, H., Hotchin, A., Bruce, L., Paterson, D. and Teale, G. (2011) 'Continuity of midwifery care and gestational weight gain in obese women: a randomised control trial', *BMC Public Health*, 11, 174, doi: 10.1186/1471-2458-11-174.

National Institute for Health and Clinical Excellence (2006) *Four Commonly Used Methods to Increase Physical Activity: Brief Interventions in Primary Care, Exercise Referral Schemes, Pedometers and Community-Based Exercise Programmes for Walking and Cycling*. London: National Institute for Health and Clinical Excellence.

National Institute for Health and Clinical Excellence (2007a) *Antenatal and Postnatal Mental Health*. London: British Psychological Society and Royal College of Psychiatrists.

National Institute for Health and Clinical Excellence (2007b) *Behaviour Change at Population, Community and Individual Level*. London: National Institute for Health and Clinical Excellence.

Neelsen, S. and Stratmann, T. (2012) 'Long-run effects of fetal influenza exposure: evidence from Switzerland', *Social Science and Medicine*, 74 (1): 58–66.

NHS Information Centre for Health and Social Care (2009) *Adult Psychiatric Morbidity in England, 2007: Results of a Household Survey*. Leeds: NHS Information Centre.

NHS Information Centre for Health and Social Care (2010) *Health Survey for England, 2009: Trend Tables*. Leeds: NHS Information Centre.

NHS Information Centre for Health and Social Care (2011) *National Diabetes Audit Mortality Analysis 2007–2008*. Leeds: NHS Information Centre.

Nilsson, M. and Emmelin, M. (2010) '"Immortal but frightened": smoking adolescents' perceptions on smoking uptake and prevention', *BMC Public Health*, 10: 776.

Nonnemaker, J.M., McNeely, C.A. and Blum, R.W. (2003) 'Public and private domains of religiosity and adolescent health risk behaviors: evidence from the National Longitudinal Study of Adolescent Health', *Social Science and Medicine*, 57 (11): 2049–54.

Norlund, S., Reuterwall, C., Höög, J., Lindah, B., Janlert, U. and Birgander, L.S. (2010) 'Burnout, working conditions and gender: results from the northern Sweden MONICA Study', *BMC Public Health*, 10: 326.

Norström, T. and Palme, J. (2010) 'Public pension institutions and old-age mortality in a comparative perspective', *International Journal of Social Welfare*, 19 (1): 121–30.

Nulman, I. (2010) 'Carbamazepine in pregnancy', *British Medical Journal*, 341: c6582.

Nunes, E.V. (2010) 'Drug use disorders among young adults: evaluation and treatment', in J.E. Grant and M.A. Potenza (eds), *Young Adult Mental Health*. New York: Oxford University Press.

Nusselder, W.J., Francom, O.H., Peeters, A. and Mackenbach, J.P. (2009) 'Living healthier for longer: comparative effects of three heart-healthy behaviors on life expectancy with and without cardiovascular disease', *BMC Public Health*, 9: 487.

Nyhlén, A., Fridell, M., Hesse, M. and Krantz, P. (2011) 'Causes of premature mortality in Swedish drug abusers: a prospective longitudinal study 1970–2006', *Journal of Forensic and Legal Medicine*, 18 (2): 66–72.

O'Brien, M. and Jack, B. (2010) 'Barriers to dying at home: the impact of poor co-ordination of community service provision for patients with cancer', *Health and Social Care in the Community*, 18 (4): 337–45.

O'Connor, T.G., Ben-Shlomo, Y., Heron, J., Golding, J., Adams, D. and Glover, V. (2005) 'Prenatal anxiety predicts individual differences in cortisol in pre-adolescent children', *Biological Psychiatry*, 58 (3): 211–17.

O'Donnell, T. (2005) 'Social class and health', in E. Denny and S. Earle (eds), *Sociology for Nurses*. Cambridge: Polity Press.

Office for National Statistics (2005) *General Household Survey 2003*. London: Her Majesty's Stationery Office.

Office for National Statistics (2006) *General Household Survey 2004*. London: Her Majesty's Stationery Office.

Office for National Statistics (2007) *General Household Survey 2005*. London: Her Majesty's Stationery Office.

Office for National Statistics (2008) *Population Estimates*. London: Her Majesty's Stationery Office.

Office for National Statistics (2009a) *Birth Statistics, England and Wales* (Series FM1), No. 37, 2008. London: Her Majesty's Stationery Office.

Office for National Statistics (2009b) *Conception Statistics, England and Wales*. London: Her Majesty's Stationery Office.

Office for National Statistics (2009c) *General Household Survey 2007*. London: Her Majesty's Stationery Office.

Office for National Statistics (2011a) *Death Registrations Summary Tables, England and Wales, 2010*. London: Her Majesty's Stationery Office.

Office for National Statistics (2011b) *General Lifestyle Survey, 2009*. London: Her Majesty's Stationery Office.

Orme, J., Powell, J., Taylor, P. and Grey, M. (eds) (2007) *Public Health for the 21st Century*. Maidenhead: Open University Press.

Orsini, N., Bellocco, R., Bottai, M., Pagano, M., Michaëlsson, K. and Wolk, A. (2008) 'Combined effects of obesity and physical activity in predicting mortality among men', *Journal of Internal Medicine*, 264 (5): 442–51.

Ortega, G., Castellà, C., Martín-Cantera, C., Ballvé, J.L., Díaz, E., Saez, M., Lozano, J., Rofes, L., Morera, C., Barceló, A., Cabezas, C., Pascual, J.A., Pérez-Ortuño, R., Saltó, E., Valverde, A. and Jané, M. (2010) 'Passive smoking in babies: the BIBE study (Brief Intervention in Babies: Effectiveness)', *BMC Public Health*, 10: 772.

Pabayo, R., Belsky, J., Gauvin, L. and Curtis, S. (2011) 'Do area characteristics predict change in moderate-to-vigorous physical activity from ages 11 to 15 years?', *Social Science and Medicine*, 72 (3): 430–8.

Padilla-Moledo, C., Castro-Piñero, J., Ortega, F.B., Mora, J., Márquez, S., Sjöström, M. and Ruiz, J.R. (2011) 'Positive health, cardiorespiratory fitness and fatness in children and adolescents', *European Journal of Public Health*, 22 (1): 52–6.

Palacios-Cena, D., Alonso-Blanco, C., Jimenez-Garcia, R., Hernandez-Barrera, V., Carrasco-Garrido, P., Pileno-Martinez, E. and Fernandez-de-las-Penas, C. (2011) 'Time trends in leisure time physical activity and physical fitness in elderly people: 20-year follow-up of the Spanish population national health survey (1987–2006)', *BMC Public Health*, 11: 799.

Palloni, A., Milesi, C., White, R. and Turner, A. (2009) 'Early childhood health, reproduction of economic inequalities and the persistence of health and mortality differentials', *Social Science and Medicine*, 68 (9): 1574–82.

Parentline Plus (2010) *When Family Life Hurts: Family Experience of Aggression in Children*. London: Family Lives Group.

Parkes, C.M., Stevenson-Hinde, J. and Marris, P. (eds) (1991) *Attachment Across the Life Cycle*. London: Routledge.

Patel, N. (2012) 'Growing old far away from home: migration, ageing and ethnicity in Europe', *Runnymede Bulletin*, Winter 2011–12 (368): 12–13.

Patsios, D. (2006) 'Pensioners, poverty and social exclusion', in C. Pantazis, D. Gordon and R. Levitas (eds), *Poverty and Social Exclusion in Britain: The Millennium Survey*. Bristol: Policy Press.

Patton, G.C., Coffey, C., Carlin, J.B., Sawyer, S.M., Williams, J., Olsson, C.A. and Wake, M. (2011) 'Overweight and obesity between adolescence and young adulthood: a 10-year prospective cohort study', *Journal of Adolescent Health*, 48 (3): 275–80.

Peadon, E., Payne, J., Henley, N., D'Antoine, H., Bartu, A., O'Leary, C., Bower, C. and Elliot, E.J. (2010) 'Women's knowledge and attitudes regarding alcohol consumption in pregnancy: a national survey', *BMC Public Health*, 10: 510.

Peebles, D.M., Marlow, N. and Brocklehurst, P. (2010) 'Antenatal magnesium sulphate', *British Medical Journal*, 341: c6004.

Peng Ng, S., Korda, R., Latz, I., Bauman, A., Bambrick, H., Liu, B., Rogers., K., Herbert, N. and Banks, E. (2011) 'Validity of self-reported height and weight and derived body mass index in middle-aged and elderly individuals in Australia', *Australian and New Zealand Journal of Public Health*, 35 (6): 557–63.

Percy, A., Wilson, J., McCartan, C. and McCrystal, P. (2011) *Teenage Drinking Cultures*. York: Joseph Rowntree Foundation.

Perry, I.J. and Lumey, L.H. (2005) 'Fetal growth and development: the role of nutrition and other factors', in D. Kuh and Y. Ben-Shlomo (eds), *A Lifecourse Approach to Chronic Disease Epidemiology*, 2nd edn. Oxford: Oxford University Press.

Pesa, J.A., Turner, L.W. and Mathews, J. (2001) 'Sex differences in barriers to contraceptive use among adolescents', *Journal of Pediatrics*, 139 (5): 689–93.

Petit, C., Chevrier, C., Durand, G., Monfort, C., Rouget, F., Garlent, R. and Cordier, S. (2010) 'Impact on fetal growth of prenatal exposure to pesticides during agricultural activities: a prospective cohort study in Brittany France', *Environmental Health*, 9: 71.

Peto, R., Lopez, A.D., Boreham, J. and Thun, M. (2010) *Mortality from Smoking in Developed Countries, 1950–2000*, 2nd edn. Oxford: Oxford University Press.

Pickard, L., Wittenberg, R., Comas-Herrera, A., King, D. and Malley, J. (2007) 'Care by spouses, care by children: projections of informal care for older people in England to 2031', *Social Policy and Society*, 6 (3): 353–66.

Pilgrim, D. (2007) *Key Concepts in Mental Health*. London: Sage.

Plant, M., Miller, P., Plant, M., Gmel, G., Kuntsche, S., Bergmark, W.K., Bloomfield, K., Csémy, L., Ozenturk, T. and Vidal, A. (2010) 'The social consequences of binge drinking among 24- to 32-year-olds in six European countries', *Substance Use and Misuse*, 45 (4): 528–42.

Platt, L. (2011) *Understanding Inequalities: Stratification and Difference*. Cambridge: Polity Press.

Pollard, M.S., Tucker, J.S., Green, H.D., Kennedy, D. and Go, M.H. (2010) 'Friendship networks and trajectories of adolescent tobacco use', *Addictive Behaviours*, 35 (7): 678–85.

Powell, J., Robison, J., Roberts, H. and Thomas, G. (2007) 'The single assessment process in primary care: older people's accounts of the process', *British Journal of Social Work*, 37 (6): 1043–58.

Priestly, M. (2010) *Disability: A Life Course Approach*. Cambridge: Polity Press.

Prins, R.G., van Empelen, P., Beenackers, M.A., Brug, J. and Oenema, A. (2010) 'Systematic development of the YouRAction program, a computer-tailored Physical Activity promotion intervention for Dutch adolescents, targeting personal motivations and environmental opportunities', *BMC Public Health*, 10: 474.

Pritchard, J. (2006) *Putting a Stop to the Abuse of Older People*. London: Help the Aged.

Quilgars, D., Searle, B. and Keung, A. (2005) Mental health and well-being', in J. Bradshaw and E. Mayhew (eds), *The Well-Being of Children in the UK*, 2nd edn. London: Save the Children Fund.

Rayner, G., Gracia, M., Young, E., Mauleon, J.R., Luque, E. and Rivera-Ferrem, M.G. (2010) 'Why are we fat? Discussions on the socioeconomic dimensions and responses to obesity', *Globalization and Health*, 6: 7.

Rees Jones, I., Papacosta, O., Whincup, P.H., Goya Wannamethee, S. and Morris, R.W. (2011) 'Class and lifestyle "lock-in" among middle-aged and older men: a Multiple Correspondence Analysis of the British Regional Heart Study', *Sociology of Health and Illness*, 33 (3): 399–419.

Regis, D. (2011) *Young People into 2011*. Exeter: Schools and Students Health Education Unit.

Reichman, N.E. and Nepomnyaschy, L. (2008) 'Maternal pre-pregnancy obesity and diagnosis of asthma in offspring at age 3 years', *Maternal and Child Health Journal*, 12 (6): 725–33.

Reilly, J.J. (2006) 'Obesity in childhood and adolescence: evidence based clinical and public health perspectives', *Postgraduate Medical Journal*, 82: 429–37.

Reynolds, A.J., Temple, J.A. and White, B.A. (2011) 'Age 26 Cost–Benefit Analysis of the Child–Parent Center Early Education Program', *Child Development*, 82 (1): 379–404.

Rice, F., Harold, G.T., Boivin, J., van den Bree, M., Hay, D.F. and Thapar, A. (2010) 'The links between prenatal stress and offspring development and psychopathology: disentangling environmental and inherited influences', *Psychological Medicine*, 40 (2): 335–42.

Rice, N.E., Lang, I.A., Henley, W. and Melzer, D. (2011) 'Common health predictors of early retirement: findings from the English Longitudinal Study of Ageing', *Age and Ageing*, 40 (1): 54–61.

Rich-Edwards, J. (2002) 'A life course approach to women's reproductive health', in D. Kuh and R. Hardy (eds), *A Life Course Approach to Women's Health*. Oxford: Oxford University Press.

Ridge, T. (2011) 'The everyday costs of poverty in childhood: a review of qualitative research exploring the lives and experiences of low-income children in the UK', *Children and Society*, 25 (1): 73–84.

Roberts, Y. (2011) 'Let's dispel this gloom about living longer and make life better for the old', *Observer*, 7 August, p. 29.

Robson, S.E. and Waugh, J. (eds) (2008) *Medical Disorders in Pregnancy: A Manual for Midwives*. Oxford: Blackwell Publishing.

Roche, K.M., Ghazarian, S.R., Little, T.D. and Leventhal, T. (2011) 'Understanding links between punitive parenting and adolescent adjustment: the relevance of context and reciprocal associations', *Journal of Research on Adolescence*, 21 (2): 448–60.

Roehr, B. (2010) 'US adolescents get a fifth of their calories from fast food, study finds', *British Medical Journal*, 341: c6406.

Rogers, A. and Pilgrim, D. (2003) *Mental Health and Inequality*. Basingstoke: Palgrave.

Rogers, A. and Pilgrim, D. (2010) *A Sociology of Mental Health and Illness*, 4th edn. Maidenhead: Open University Press.

Rogers, L. (2010) 'Test-tube babies may inherit fertility problems', *Sunday Times*, 7 February, p. 4.

Rostosky, S.S., Danner, F. and Riggle, E.D.B. (2007) 'Is religiosity a protective factor against substance use in young adulthood? Only if you're straight!', *Journal of Adolescent Health*, 40 (5): 440–7.

Royal College of Psychiatrists (2010) *No Health without Public Mental Health: The Case for Action*. London: Royal College of Psychiatrists.

Ruckstuhl, K., Colijn, G.P., Amiot, V. and Vinish, E. (2010) 'Mother's occupation and sex ratio at birth', *BMC Public Health*, 10: 269.

Rugg, J. (2010) *Young People and Housing: The Need for a New Policy Agenda*. York: Joseph Rowntree Foundation.

Ruidavets, J.-B., Ducimetière, P., Evans, A., Montaye, M., Haas, B., Bingham, A., Yarnell, J., Amouyel, P., Arveiler, D., Kee, F., Bongard, V. and Ferrières, J. (2010) 'Patterns of alcohol consumption and ischaemic heart disease in culturally divergent countries: the Prospective Epidemiological Study of Myocardial Infarction (PRIME)', *British Medical Journal*, 341: c6077.

Rutger, C.M.E. and van den Eijnden, R. (2007) 'Substance use in adolescence', in J. Coleman, L. Hendry and M. Kloep (eds), *Adolescence and Health*. Chichester: John Wiley and Sons Ltd.

Sainsbury Centre for Mental Health: Rethink (2010) *The Diversion Dividend: Interim Report*. London: Sainsbury Centre for Mental Health: Rethink.

Salonen, M.K., Kajantie, E., Osmond, C., Forsen, T., Yliharsila, H., Paile-Hyvarinen, M., Barker, D.J.P. and Eriksosn, G. (2010) 'Prenatal and childhood growth and leisure time physical activity in adult life', *European Journal of Public Health*, 21 (6): 719–24.

Sanders, C., Donovan, J. and Dieppe, P. (2002) 'The significance and consequences of having painful and disabled joints in older age: co-existing accounts of normal and disrupted biographies', *Sociology of Health and Illness*, 24 (2): 227–53.

Sanderson, K., Patton, G.C., McKercher, C., Dwyer, T. and Venn, A.J. (2011) 'Overweight and obesity in childhood and risk of mental disorder: a 20-year cohort study', *Australian and New Zealand Journal of Psychiatry*, 45 (5): 384–92.

Sandman, C.A., Glynn, L.M., Dunkel Schetter, C., Wadhwa, P.D., Garite, T.J., Chicz-DeMet, A. and Hobel, C.J. (2006) 'Elevated maternal cortisol early in pregnancy predicts third trimester levels of placental corticotropin-releasing hormone in pregnant women: priming the placental clock', *Peptides*, 21 (6): 1457–63.

Sassler, S. (2010) 'Partnering across the life course: sex, relationships, and mate selection', *Journal of Marriage and Family*, 72 (3): 557–75.

Sauber-Schatz, E.K., Markovic, N., Weiss, H.B., Bodnar, L.M., Wilson, J.W. and Pearlman, M.D. (2010) 'Descriptive epidemiology of birth trauma in the United States in 2003', *Paediatric and Perinatal Epidemiology*, 24 (2): 116–24.

Schmidt, M., Absalah, S., Nierkens, V. and Stronks, K. (2008) 'Which factors engage women in deprived neighbourhoods to participate in exercise referral schemes', *BMC Public Health*, 8: 371.

Schneider, B., Grebner, K., Schnabel, A., Hampel, H., Georgi, K. and Seidler, A. (2011) 'Impact of employment status and work-related factors on risk of completed suicide: a case-control psychological autopsy study', *Psychiatry Research*, 190 (2–3): 265–70.

Scholtens, S., Brunekreef, B., Visscher, T.L.S., Smit, H.A., Kerkhof, M., de Jongste, J.C., Gerritsen, J. and Wijga, A.H. (2007) 'Reported versus measured body weight and height of 4-year-old children and the prevalence of overweight', *European Journal of Public Health*, 17 (4): 369–74.

Schuckit, M.A. (2009) 'Alcohol-use disorders', *The Lancet*, 373: 492–501.

Scott, E.J., Dimairo, M., Hind, D., Goyder, E., Copeland, R.J., Breckon, J.D., Crank, H., Walters, S.J., Loban, A. and Cooper, C.L. (2011) '"Booster" interventions to sustain increases in physical activity in middle-aged adults in deprived urban neighbourhoods: internal pilot and feasibility study', *BMC Public Health*, 11: 129.

Sealy, Y.M. (2010) 'Parents' perceptions of food availability; implications for childhood obesity', 49 (6): 565–80.

Seaman, P. and Ikegwuonu, T. (2010) *Young People and Alcohol: Influences on How they Drink*. York: Joseph Rowntree Foundation.

Sellström, E., Bremberg, S. and O'Campo, P. (2010) 'Yearly incidence of mental disorders in economically inactive young adults', *European Journal of Public Health*, 21 (6): 812–14.

Senior, J. (2010) 'All joy and no fun: why parents hate parenting', *New York Magazine*, 4 July, p. 15.

Sharif, N., Brown, W. and Rutter, D. (2008) *Systematic Map Report 3: The Extent and Impact of Depression on BME Older People and the Acceptability and Effectiveness of Social Care Provision*. London: Social Care Institute for Excellence.

Shrewsbury, V. and Wardle, J. (2008) 'Socioeconomic status and adiposity in childhood: a systematic review of cross-sectional studies 1990–2005', *Obesity*, 16 (2): 275–84.

Sjögren, K., Ekvall Hansson, E. and Stjernberg, L. (2011) 'Parenthood and factors that influence outdoor recreational physical activity from a gender perspective', *BMC Public Health*, 11: 93.

Sloan, F., Grossman, D. and Platt, A. (2011) 'Heavy episodic drinking in early adulthood and outcomes in midlife', *Journal of Studies on Alcohol and Drugs*, 72 (3): 459–70.

Smith, A.E. and Krishnan-Sarin, S. (2010). 'Tobacco use and nicotine dependence', in J.E. Grant and M.A. Potenza (eds), *Young Adult Mental Health*. New York: Oxford University Press.

Social Exclusion Unit (2005) *Excluded Older People: Social Exclusion Unit Interim Report*. London: Office of the Deputy Prime Minister, Her Majesty's Stationery Office.

SomnIA (2010) *Optimising Quality of Sleep Among Older People in the Community and Care Homes: An Integrated Approach*. Guildford: SomnIA.

Sona, A., Maggiani, G., Astengo, M., Comba, M., Chiusano, V., Isaia, G., Merlo, C., Pricop, L., Quagliotti, E., Moiraghi, C., Fonte, G. and Bo, M. (2012) 'Determinants of recourse to hospital treatment in the elderly', *European Journal of Public Health*, 22 (1): 76–80.

Sondhi, A. and Turner, C. (2011) *The Influence of Family and Friends on Young People's Drinking*. York: Joseph Rowntree Foundation.

Sørensen, H.J., Mortensen, E.L., Reinisch, J.M. and Mednick, S.A. (2011) 'A prospective study of smoking in young women and risk of later psychiatric hospitalization', *Nordic Journal of Psychiatry*, 65 (1): 3–8.

Spencer, N. (2001) 'The social patterning of teenage pregnancy', *Journal of Epidemiological Community Health*, 55 (5): 1–5.

Spiegel, K., Leproult, R. and Van Cauter, E. (1999) 'Impact of sleep debt on metabolic and endocrine function', *The Lancet*, 354 (9188): 1435–9.

Spijkers, W., Jansen, D.E.M.C. and Reijneveld, S.A. (2011) 'The impact of area deprivation on parenting stress', *European Journal of Public Health*, doi: 10.1093/eurpub/ckr146.

Steeman, E., Godderis, J., Grypdonck, M., De Bal, N. and de Casterle, B.D. (2007) 'Living with dementia from the perspective of older people: is it a positive story?', *Aging and Mental Health*, 11 (2): 119–30.

Stegeman, I., Otte-Trojel, T., Costongs, C. and Considine, J. (2012) *Health and Active Aging*. Brussels: Eurohealthnet.

Stein, Z., Susser, M., Saenger, G. and Marolla, F. (1975) *Famine and Human Development: The Dutch Hunger Winter of 1944–45*. New York: Oxford University Press.

Steinberg, J. (2001) 'We know some things: parent–adolescent relationships in retrospect and prospect', *Journal of Research on Adolescence*, 11 (1): 1–19.

Strang-Karlsson, S., Räikkönen, K., Pesonen, A.-K., Kajantie, E., Paavonen, E.J., Lahti, J., Hovi, P. and Andersson, S. (2008) 'Very low birth weight and behavioral symptoms of attention deficit hyperactivity disorder in young adulthood: the Helsinki study of very-low-birth-weight adults', *American Journal of Psychiatry*, 165 (10): 1345–53.

Suvisaari, J., Aalto-Setälä, T., Tuulio-Henriksson, A., Härkänen, T., Saarni, S.I., Perälä, J., Schreck, M. and Lönnqvist, J. (2009) 'Mental disorders in young adulthood', *Psychological Medicine*, 39 (2): 287–99.

Sweeney, M.M. (2010) 'Remarriage and stepfamilies: strategic sites for family scholarship in the 21st century', *Journal of Marriage and Family*, 72 (3): 667–84.

Sweeting, H., West, P., Young, R. and Der, G. (2010) 'Can we explain increases in young people's psychological distress over time?', *Social Science and Medicine*, 71 (10): 1819–30.

Swinburn, B.A., Sacks, G., Hall, K.D., McPherson, K., Finegood, D.T., Moodie, M.L. and Gortmaker, S.L. (2011) 'The global obesity pandemic: shaped by global drivers and local environments', *The Lancet*, 378 (9793): 804–14.

Szinovacz, M.E. and Davey, A. (2006) 'Effects of retirement and grandchild care on depressive symptoms', *International Journal of Aging and Human Development*, 62 (1): 1–20.

Tanaka, K., Miyake, Y., Arakawa, M., Sasaki, S. and Ohya, Y. (2010) 'Household smoking and dental caries in schoolchildren: the Ryukyus Child Health Study', *BMC Public Health*, 10: 335.

Tassitano, R.M., Barros, M.V.G., Tenorio, M.C.M., Bezerra, J., Florindo, A.A., Reis, R.S. (2010) 'Enrollment in physical education is associated with health-related behavior among high school students', *Journal of School Health*, 80 (3): 126–33.

Taylor, D.H., Kuchibhatla, M., Østbye, T., Plassman, B.L. and Clipp, E.C. (2008) 'The effect of spousal caregiving and bereavement on depressive symptoms', *Aging and Mental Health*, 12 (1): 100–7.

Thomson, J.A., Wang, W.C., Browning, C. and Kendig, H.L. (2010) 'Self-reported medication side effects in an older cohort living independently in the community – the Melbourne Longitudinal Study on Healthy Ageing (MELSHA): cross-sectional analysis of prevalence and risk factors', *BMC Geriatrics*, 10: 37.

Timimi, S. (2004) 'Rethinking childhood depression', *British Medical Journal*, 329: 1394–6.

Torp, S., Nielsen, R.A., Fosså, S.D., Gudbergsson, S.B. and Dahl, A.A. (2012) 'Change in employment status of 5-year cancer survivors', *European Journal of Public Health*, doi: 10.1093/eurpub/ckr192.

Treasure, J. and Friederich, H.C. (2009) 'Neural correlates of impaired cognitive-behavioural flexibility in anorexia-nervosa', *American Journal of Psychiatry*, 166: 608–16.

Tromp, K., Claessens, J.J.M., Knijnenburg, S.L., van der Pal, H.J.H., van Leeuwen, F.E., Caron, H.N., Beerendonk, C.C.M. and Kremer, L.C.M. (2011) 'Reproductive status in adult male long-term survivors of childhood cancer', *Human Reproduction*, 26 (7): 1775–83.

Tucker-Seeley, R.D., Li, Y., Sorensen, G. and Subramanian, S.V. (2011) 'Lifecourse socioeconomic circumstances and multimorbidity among older adults', *BMC Public Health*, 11: 313.

Umberson, D., Pudrovska, T. and Reczek, C. (2010) 'Parenthood, childlessness, and well-being: a life course perspective', *Journal of Marriage and Family*, 72 (30): 612–29.

United Nations Children's Fund (UNICEF) (2007) *Child Poverty in Perspective: An Overview of Child Well-Being in Rich Countries, Innocenti Report Card 7*. Florence: United Nations Children's Fund Innocenti Research Centre.

United Nations Children's Fund (UNICEF) (2010) *The Children Left Behind. A League Table of Inequality in Child Wellbeing in the World's Rich Countries*. Florence: United Nations Children's Fund Innocenti Research Centre.

United Nations Children's Fund (UNICEF) (2011a) *Child Well-Being in the UK, Spain and Sweden*. London: United Nations Children's Fund and IPSOS Mori.

United Nations Children's Fund (UNICEF) (2011b) *The State of the World's Children 2011*. New York: United Nations Children's Fund.

Valentine, G., Jayne, M. and Gould, M. (2010) *Alcohol Consumption and Family Life*. York: Joseph Rowntree Foundation.

Van den Bergh, B.R.H. and Marcoen, A. (2004) 'High antenatal maternal anxiety is related to ADHD symptoms, externalizing problems, and anxiety in 8- and 9-year-olds', *Child Development*, 75 (4): 1085–97.

van der Wel, K.A. (2011) 'Long-term effects of poor health on employment: the significance of life stage and educational level', *Sociology of Health and Illness*, 33 (7): 1096–1111.

van Dijk, A.E., van Eijsden, M., Strionks, K., Gemke, R.J.B.J. and Vrijkotte, T.G.M. (2010) 'Cardio-metabolic risk in 5-year-old children prenatally exposed to maternal psychosocial stress: the ABCD study', *BMC Public Health*, 10: 251.

Van Rossem, R., Berten, H. and Van Tuyckom, C. (2010) 'AIDS knowledge and sexual activity among Flemish secondary school students: a multilevel analysis of the effects of type of education', *BMC Public Health*, 10: 30.

van Solinge, H. and Henkens, K. (2010) 'Living longer, working longer? The impact of subjective life expectancy on retirement intentions and behavior', *European Journal of Public Health*, 20 (1): 47–51.

VanderWeele, T.J., Lantos, J.D. and Lauderdale, D.S. (2012) 'Rising preterm birth rates, 1989–2004: changing demographics or changing obstetric practice?', *Social Science and Medicine*, 74 (2): 196–201.

Vederhus, B.J., Markestad, T., Eide, G.E., Graue, M. and Halvorsen, T. (2010) 'Health-related quality of life after extremely preterm birth: a matched controlled cohort study', *Health and Quality of Life Outcomes*, 8: 53.

Venn, S. and Arber, S. (2011) 'Day-time sleep and active ageing in later life', *Ageing and Society*, 31 (2): 197–216.

Venter, K. (2011) 'Fathers "care" too: the impact of family relationships on the experience of work for parents of disabled children', *Sociological Research Online*, 16 (3). Available at: www.socresonline.org.uk/16/3/1.html.

Vera-Sanso, P. (2006) 'Experiences in old age: a South Indian example of how functional age is socially structured', *Oxford Development Studies*, 34 (4): 457–72.

Victor, C. (2010) *Ageing, Health and Care*. Bristol: Policy Press.

Victor, C., Scrambler, S. and Bond, J. (2009) *Growing Older*. Maidenhead: McGraw-Hill.

Vincent, J.A. (2003) *Old Age*. London: Routledge.

Vincent, J.A. (2006) 'Age and old age', in G. Payne (ed.), *Social Divisions*. Basingstoke: Macmillan.

Wadhwa, P.D., Culhane, J., Rauh, V. and Barve, S.S. (2001) 'Stress and preterm birth: neuroendocrine, immune-inflammatory and vascular mechanisms', *Maternal and Child Health Journal*, 5 (2): 119–25.

Wadhwa, P.D., Sandman, C.A., Porto, M., Dunkel-Schetter, C. and Garite, T.J. (1993) 'The association between prenatal stress and infant birth weight and gestational age at birth: a prospective investigation', *American Journal of Obstetrics and Gynaecology*, 169 (4): 858–65.

Wadsworth, M.E. and Compas, B.E. (2002) 'Coping with family conflict and economic strain: the adolescent perspective', *Journal of Research on Adolescence*, 12 (2): 243–74.

Walker, M. (2006) *Breastfeeding Management for the Clinician: Using the Evidence*. Sudbury, MA: Jones and Bartlett Publishers, Inc.

Walton, A. and Flouri, E. (2010) 'Contextual risk, maternal parenting and adolescent externalizing behaviour problems: the role of emotion regulation', *Child: Care, Health and Development*, 36 (2): 275–84.

Ward, L.M. and Friedman, K. (2006) 'Using TV as a guide: associations between television viewing and adolescents' sexual attitudes and behavior', *Journal of Research on Adolescence*, 16 (1): 133–56.

West, R., Zatonski, W., Przewozniak, K. and Jarvis M.J. (2007) 'Can we trust national smoking prevalence figures? Discrepancies between biochemically assessed and self-reported smoking rates in three countries', *Cancer Epidemiology, Biomarkers and Prevention*, 16 (4): 820–2.

Westerlund, H., Vahtera, J., Ferrie, J.E., Singh-Manoux, A., Pentti, J., Melchior, M., Leineweber, C., Jokela, M., Siegrist, J., Goldberg, M., Zuins, M. and Kivimäki, M. (2010) 'Effect of retirement on major chronic conditions and fatigue: French GAZEL occupational cohort study', *British Medical Journal*, 341: c6149.

Wheeler, S.B. (2010) 'Effects of self-esteem and academic performance on adolescent decision-making: an examination of early sexual intercourse and illegal substance use', *Journal of Adolescent Health*, 47 (6): 582–90.

Wiencke, J.K., Thurston, S.W., Kelsey, K.T., Varkonyi, A., Wain, J.C., Mark, E.J. and Christiani, D.C. (1999) 'Early age at smoking initiation and tobacco carcinogen DNA damage in the lung', *Journal of National Cancer Institute*, 91 (7): 614–19.

Wijga, A.H., Scholtens, S., Bemelmans, W.J.E., de Jongste, J.C., Kerkhof, N., Schipper, M., Sanders, E.A., Gerritsen, J., Brunekreef, B. and Smit, H.A. (2010) 'Comorbidities of obesity in school children: a cross-sectional study in the PIAMA birth cohort', *BMC Public Health*, 10: 184.

Wilkinson, K., Martin, I.C., Gough, M.J., Stewart, J.A.D., Lucas, S.B., Freeth, H., Bull, B. and Mason, M. (2010) *An Age-Old Problem: A Review of the Care Received by Elderly Patients Undergoing Surgery*. London: National Confidential Enquiry into Patient Outcome and Death.

Williams, A., Ylanne, V. and Wadleigh, P.M. (2007) 'Selling the "elixir of life": images of the elderly in an *Olivio* advertising campaign', *Journal of Aging Studies*, 21 (1): 1–21.

Wills, T. A. (2008) 'Adolescent health and health behaviours.' *International Encyclopaedia of Public Health*, 105–12, doi: 10.1016/B0-08043076-7/03848-1.

Wilson, H.W. and Widom, C.S. (2011) 'Pathways from childhood abuse and neglect to HIV-risk sexual behavior in middle adulthood', *Journal of Consulting and Clinical Psychology*, 79 (2): 236–46.

World Health Organization (WHO) (1946) *Preamble to the Constitution of the World Health Organization*. Geneva: World Health Organization.

World Health Organization (WHO) (1986) *Ottawa Charter for Health Promotion*. Copenhagen: World Health Organization Regional Office for Europe.

World Health Organization (WHO) (2002) *Active Ageing: A Policy Framework*. Geneva: World Health Organization.

World Health Organization (WHO), World Bank, United Nations Children's Fund (UNICEF) and United Nations Population Fund (2010) *Trends in Maternal Mortality: 1990 to 2008*. Geneva: World Health Organization.

Xu, W.L., Atti, A.R., Gatz, M., Pedersen, N.L., Johansson, B. and Fratiglioni, L. (2011) 'Midlife overweight and obesity increase late-life dementia risk: a population-based twin study', *Neurology*, 76 (8): 1568–74.

Yeandle, S., Bennett, C., Buckner, L., Fry, G. and Price, C. (2007) *Diversity in Caring: Towards Equality for Carers*. London: Carers UK.

Zarate, C.A. (2010) 'Psychiatric disorders in young adults: depression assessment and treatment', in J.E. Grant and M.A. Potenza (eds), *Young Adult Mental Health*. New York: Oxford University Press.

Zarrit, S.H. (1996) 'Continuities and discontinuities in very late life', in V.I. Bengston (ed.), *Adulthood and Aging: Research on Continuities and Discontinuities*. New York: Springer.

Zhang, Z. and Hayward, M.D. (2006) 'Gender, the marital life course, and cardiovascular disease in late midlife', *Journal of Marriage and Family*, 68 (3): 639–57.

Zimmermann, E., Holst, C. and Sørensen, T.I. (2011) 'Morbidity, including fatal morbidity, throughout life in men entering adult life as obese', *PLoS One*, 6 (4): 1–7.

Zunzunegui, M.-V., Béland, F., Sanchez, M.-T. and Otero, A. (2009) 'Longevity and relationships with children: the importance of the parental role', *BMC Public Health*, 9: 351.

Index

Glossary terms are shown in **bold**.